GCSE Home Economics

FOOD FOR HEALTH

Dodie Roe

Longman

Longman Group UK Limited
Longman House, Burnt Mill, Harlow, Essex CM20 2JE, England
and Associated Companies throughout the world

First published 1986
Third impression 1987
Set in 10/12 point Palatino

Printed in Great Britain
by Scotprint Limited, Musselburgh, Scotland

ISBN 0-582-22479-9

The books in this series

Families and Child Development by Sharon Goodyer

Food for Health by Dodie Roe

Home and Consumer by Dodie Roe

Textiles for People by Maureen Wilkinson

Dodie Roe is also Series editor.

The following topics relevant to this book are covered in other titles in the series.

Families and Child Development

Topic	Information available
Food and drink	Diet and food for babies, children and pregnant women.

Home and Consumer

Topic	Information available
Consumer information	Descriptions of organisations providing information, and how to get help and advice as a consumer.
Consumer protection	The laws relating to the consumer.
First aid	How to treat simple kitchen injuries.
Furnishings	Includes a survey of different floor and wall coverings available.
Kitchen planning	Choosing what items are needed and where to position them.
Safety	Causes of and statistics on accidents in the kitchen. Laws.
Shopping	Different types of shops and ways of buying foods.

Contents

Preface

This book is one of a series of four, written particularly to help teachers interpret and pupils succeed in the GCSE examination courses in Home Economics. The authors have worked together on developing a problem solving approach and have tried out ideas in the classroom. The other books in the series are:

Families and Child Development
Home and Consumer
Textiles for People

What is so special about this examination?

One of the aims of the GCSE examination course is to develop the skills of decision making, which are necessary throughout life. It also aims to help individuals to lead effective lives, as members of the family and community, and to provide them with the management skills to use resources wisely and to recognise the interrelationship between the need for food, clothing, shelter and security.

What does this approach entail?

The authors of these books have used the subject matter of Home Economics to provide pupils with opportunities to:

– identify needs in a particular area;
– recall, seek out and apply knowledge relevant to the situation;
– identify ways of carrying out a task or solving a problem, isolating the priorities;
– decide upon and plan a course of action;
– carry out a course of action;
– evaluate the effectiveness of the course of action.

It is hoped that if pupils are able to develop decision making skills they will be able to recall and apply these criteria in different situations.

Food for Health is a book for pupils, designed to provide course work in the food area of the GCSE syllabus. It provides recipes which reflect current nutritional thinking, and seeks to help pupils to relate food and health, to appreciate the consumer aspects, and to consider the aesthetic elements of food.

Dodie Roe
Series editor

About using this book

You may think that this is just another recipe book, but it is different in two important ways.

– The recipes are especially chosen to help you to eat a more healthy diet. You will find out more about why this is necessary in Chapter 1.
– It provides you with the opportunity for making *decisions* about your choice of foods.

You may not always be in a position to choose the food you eat – it may be cooked for you. But there will probably be some times, perhaps at school lunch time or when you eat out, when you will have to decide for yourself, and sooner or later you may be responsible for choosing food for someone else.

How are you going to decide what to choose? Will it always be chips just because *you* like them? Will having bought pies all the time do your family any harm? Does it matter if you never eat fresh vegetables?

Making decisions

This book will help you to make decisions about food. Every time you have to make a decision about choosing food you will need to consider:

1   Who is this meal or dish for? Is it for one person, or a group of people? What special needs will they have, for example are they very young and still growing, or elderly with digestion problems, or are there any foods they cannot eat? In Chapters 2, 16 and 19 you will find more information about people's special needs for food.

Will there be any special difficulties such as not having much time or lack of money? (See Chapter 2.)
2   What will you have to think about when choosing and preparing food? For example will the meal be a healthy choice and provide variety? (See Chapter 1.)

You will also need to think about making food attractive for other people – is there a variety of colour, texture, flavours?

Have you considered the cost, the time you have? Have you any equipment you could use to help save time or effort, for example a food mixer?

(See Chapter 2 for more information.)
3   What are the alternatives: making everything yourself, buying food ready made, or using some convenience foods with fresh ingredients?

Which ingredients should you choose? You may need to experiment, e.g. try making pastry with different types of fat to see which is the most acceptable, or compare convenience foods with fresh ones to see which look and taste better, which is the most expensive etc.
4   How you are going to set about the task of preparing a dish or meal? This will mean planning your use of time, money, equipment, food etc.
5   Actually carrying out the task. Remember, as well as all the things listed above, you will need to make the food look and taste good. There are lots of suggestions in the book for adding

flavour and making food look attractive.

6   How you will know that you have made the right decision?

The food may look all right, but is 'the proof of the pudding in the eating'? Obviously food must look and taste good, but it should help to keep you healthy too. How can you tell if it does?

To provide a healthy diet you should be sure to have a variety of foods and nutrients. To find out which nutrients there are in your foods you could look up the foods in a book, or use one of the computer programs on the right. You could also use the table on page 11 to help you to see if you have shown a good knowledge of nutrition, made an economical choice of time, money, fuel and equipment, chosen dishes which look and taste attractive, and shown that you are able to carry out the choice, preparation and serving of food.

These are your decisions pages. As you will need to return to them often there is a grey line down their outside edges so you can pick them out easily. Each time you prepare and cook a dish or meal check through the list numbered 1–6.

Computer programs which analyse foods for nutrients

Microdiet (BBC or RML) Longman Microsoftware, 62 Hallfield Road, Layerthorpe, York Y03 7XQ.

Balance Your Diet (BBC or RML) Cambridge Microsoftware, The Edinburgh Building, Shaftesbury Road, Cambridge CB2 2RU

Nupack (RML) ILEA, ILECC, Bethwin Road, London SE5 OPQ

More information about nutrition and digestion may be obtained from *Eat to live*, Dodie Roe, Longman (1983).

Acknowledgements

We are grateful to the following for permission to reproduce photographs:

Creda, 2.3; *Farmers Weekly*, 8.28 and 8.29 (photo Charles Topham); Harbenware, 3.12; Philips Electronics, 3.20; Picturepoint, 8.27; Prestige, 3.7; Tefal, 2.4, 3.16 and 3.17.
All other photographs including the colour sections by Longman Photographic Unit.

Cover illustration by Andrew Aloof and Associates

1 Introduction

Food and our health

If we eat a wide variety of foods, but not too much of anything, and take some exercise we will probably stay healthy. However, most of us choose the food we *like* rather than the food which is good for our health, and this is why some people suffer from the diseases which could have been avoided with a sensible diet. For example:

1 Too many sweet foods and poor teeth cleaning can cause tooth decay, and gum disease.
2 Too much fat can make us overweight and may cause heart disease.
3 Too much salt can cause high blood pressure which could lead to a heart attack and strokes.
4 Too little fibre can cause bowel diseases and cancer.

Nutrients

All foods are made up of nutrients, but unfortunately no one food contains all the nutrients we need to keep alive. We need to eat a variety of foods in order to make sure we have some of all the nutrients the body needs.

There is a summary of the most important nutrients that the body needs, and some of the foods which provide them, in the table on page 5. **Nutrition** is knowing about which foods to eat and how the body uses food. (More information about nutrition may be found in *Eat to Live*.*)

It is not always easy to remember which nutrients there are in every food, but if you eat foods from each of the groups in Figure 1.1 regularly you should have all the nutrients the body needs.

Fibre and water

We also need **Fibre** and **Water**. These are not nutrients, but are very important for the body.

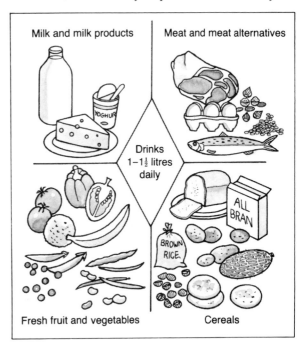

Figure 1.1

* Dodie Roe, *Eat to Live*, Longman, 1983.

Fibre

This makes us feel full, speeds up the passage of foods through the body and research suggests that it may help prevent diseases such as bowel diseases, gall stones, gastric ulcers and coronary heart disease. Fibre is found in wholemeal flour and bread, dried fruits, berry fruits, potatoes (especially the skins), nuts, peas, beans, sweetcorn and bran cereals.

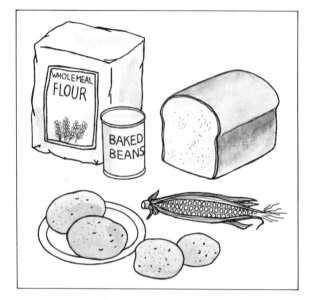

Figure 1.2   Foods containing fibre

Most people would benefit by *eating 25% more fibre*. This means eating 30 g a day. Because this would probably mean eating more starchy carbohydrate foods it would be necessary to take some exercise to avoid putting on weight.

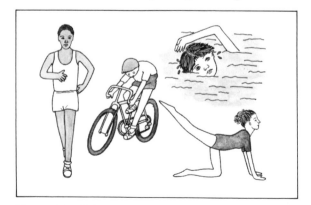

Figure 1.3   Taking exercise

Water

About 70% of the body's weight is water. Water is lost in perspiration and must be replaced. *At least one litre of non-alcoholic liquid should be drunk daily* (one and a half litres for adults). Even more than this may be needed in hot climates and in hot weather. This can be as tea, coffee, squash, or other drinks as well as just water. We can last several weeks without food, but we would only last a few days without water. Alcoholic drinks do not help because they cause the body to lose water.

Improving our diet

Unfortunately we do not always eat as varied a diet as we could. In particular many people eat too much sugar, fat, and salt and eat too little fibre.

Too much sugar

This can harm teeth and lead to weight problems, heart disease and diabetes. We can eat less by cutting out sugar in tea, coffee and other milk drinks, sweets, chocolates, ice cream, jams, fizzy drinks, convenience foods and baked foods like cakes and biscuits. Most people could *eat 10% less sugar*.

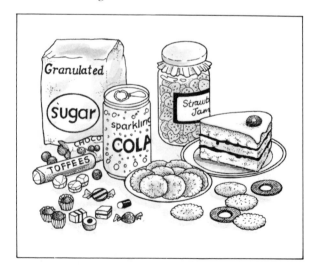

Figure 1.4   Foods high in sugar

Too much fat

This can make us overweight and cause heart trouble. A large amount of the fat we eat comes from animal sources, e.g. dairy products, meat, lard. This fat is called **saturated fat** and it can increase the amount of **cholesterol** (a fatty substance found in the blood stream) leading to blockage of the arteries and heart disease. **Polyunsaturated fats** contain some of the essential fats the body needs and it is thought tha they can help to reduce the cholesterol in your blood. They are found in most vegetable oils and fats and some fish. Most people could *eat less fat* by avoiding fried foods, cakes, pastries, cream, butter, cheese (except cottage or low fat cheeses), processed foods and full cream milk.

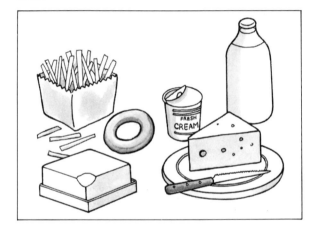

Figure 1.5 Fatty foods

To change saturated fats for polyunsaturated fats we could use margarine high in polyunsaturates for spreading and baking, use vegetable oil for frying and for salad dressings, include some oily fish in the diet, e.g. fresh or smoked mackerel, herrings, kippers, salmon, tuna, sardines.

Too much salt

Salt can accumulate in the body if the heart or kidneys are not working properly. High salt intakes may lead to high blood pressure which can lead to heart attacks. Most people could *eat 10% less salt* by using less in cooking, avoiding processed foods or leaving salt off the table.

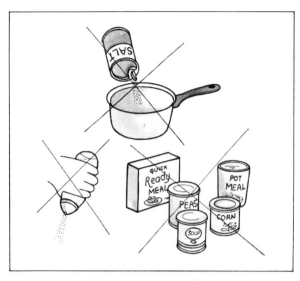

Figure 1.6 Eating less salt

Dietary goals

The changes to our eating patterns mentioned above are sometimes referred to as the **dietary goals**,* or what we should be aiming for when eating. The Dietary Goals are to:

1 Cut down sugar. 4 Increase fibre.
2 Cut down fat. 5 Eat a *variety* of foods
3 Cut down salt.   and take more exercise.

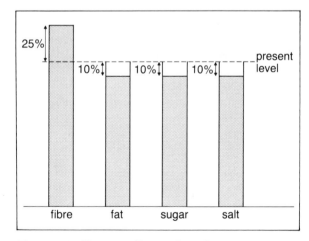

Figure 1.7 How our diet needs to change

* To read more about the dietary goals see the NACNE report (National Advisory Council for Nutrition Education), *Proposals for Nutritional Guidelines for Health Education in Britain*, Health Education Council, 1983.

Table 1.1   Recipes for fruit (apple) crumble

Traditional recipe	Adapted recipe	Changes
Filling 600 g cooking apples	600 g cooking apples	
75 g sugar	50 g sugar	Less sugar
Crumble topping 150 g plain white flour	100 g wholemeal flour 50 g mixed chopped nuts 50 g porridge oats	More fibre More fibre More fibre
75 g butter or margarine	30 g polyunsaturated margarine	Less saturated fat
50 g granulated sugar	25 g demerara sugar	Less sugar

Recipes in this book

The recipes in this book have, where possible, been chosen to help you to meet the dietary goals. For example:

1   Wholemeal flour has been used instead of white.

2   Salt has been reduced or left out and other flavourings used.

3   Grilling and baking have been chosen as cooking methods in preference to frying or roasting.

4   Skimmed milk has been used instead of full fat milk.

5   Low fat cheese has been used instead of high fat cheese.

6   Frying of vegetables has been left out when making casseroles.

7   The amount of sugar used has been cut down where possible.

For example, the table above shows a traditional recipe compared with the adapted version given in this book.

Some ideas for you to try

1   Find recipes in another book for some of the dishes in this book. Make a chart like the one in the table above to show the changes that have been made. Put a star by the side of the most important ones.

2   Keep a record of the dishes you find, either in this book or any other, which will help you to reach the dietary goals. Make a chart like the table below which you can fill in and tick off for each recipe.

Table 1.2

Recipe	Book	Page	High fibre	Low salt	Low sugar	Low fat

Table 1.3 The most important nutrients the body needs, and some foods which provide them

Minerals

Needed for	Nutrient	Found in
Building teeth and bones; helping the blood to clot after injury	Calcium and phosphorus	Milk, cheese, flour, cabbage, eggs, fish bones.
Making haemoglobin in the red blood cells	Iron	Liver, corned beef, meat, baked beans, curry powder, eggs, dried fruits, cabbage, chocolate, black treacle
Replacing the salt lost in perspiration	Sodium chloride (salt)	Table salt, salty foods e.g. bacon, cheese
Strengthening teeth against decay	Fluoride	Water (depends on where you live), tea, sea-water fish
Making the hormone thyroxine produced by the thyroid gland	Iodine	Sea foods, milk, green vegetables, water

Vitamins

Needed for	Nutrient	Found in
Healthy sight and skin, stopping infection, healing wounds	A (Retinol and carotene)	Margarine, sardines, apricots, fruit, vegetables
Healthy nerves, skin, muscles; to help the body use foods which provide energy	B1 (Thiamin)	Wholemeal bread, Marmite, eggs, pork, green vegetables
For growth, health of eyes and mouth; for the release of energy from food	B2 (Riboflavin)	Marmite, liver, green vegetables, beer, peanuts
Making red blood cells	B12 (Cobalamin)	Liver
Cell growth particularly during pregnancy	Folic acid	Green leafy vegetables
To help the body use energy from food.	Nicotinic acid	Marmite, liver, kidney, beef, pork
For healthy gums and skin; to help stop infection and heal wounds	C (Ascorbic acid)	Fruit, especially citrus fruits, green vegetables, tomatoes
To enable the body to absorb the calcium needed for forming bones and teeth	D (Cholecalciferol)	Margarine, butter, oily fish, eggs, cheese, sunlight

Protein, carbohydrate, fats

Needed for	Nutrient	Found in
Building and repair of the body tissues	Protein	Meat, fish, eggs, cheese, peas, beans, lentils, soya, nuts, bread
Energy (all foods provide energy but we should try to get most from the starchy carbohydrates as protein is an expensive source and too much fat should be avoided)	Carbohydrate (a) starch (b) sugar	Flour, rice, pasta, potatoes, cereals Sugar, jam, syrup, chocolate, biscuits, tinned foods
Surrounding and protecting the vital organs, e.g. the kidneys and the skeleton; provides the fat-soluble vitamins A and D	Fats	Butter, lard, margarine, oil, fat on meat, milk, cheese, chocolate

3 On food labels there is a list of the
   ingredients. These are in order with the one
   there is most of at the top.

INGREDIENTS: Tomatoes, wheat flour,
sugar, salt, vegetable oil and spices

Figure 1.8   Food label from tinned soup

   Make a label like the one in Figure 1.8 for
   some of the dishes in this book.
4 Collect food labels from packets and tins.
   Sort them into groups:
   (a)   those with no additives, preservatives or
         artificial flavourings;
   (b)   those which should go on a *black list*
         because they are very high in artificial
         additives;
   (c)   those with a moderate amount of
         additives which could be eaten
         occasionally.
5 Make a high fibre, low sugar or low salt
   recipe leaflet yourself which would help
   others to meet the dietary goals. Do not
   forget to explain why it is important.

2 Meal planning

When you are putting a meal together you will need to think about the dietary goals (see chapter 1). Try to include a variety of foods over the whole day without too much fat, sugar or salt. Make sure you include some foods which contain fibre.

Special needs

Some people may have special needs.

Pregnant women

What a mother eats before a baby is born can affect the health of her baby. It is not necessary to eat for two — in fact a woman is likely to become overweight if she does. It is important to eat enough foods containing calcium and iron because these will be taken from the mother to make the baby grow. Plenty of fruit and fibrous foods should be eaten to prevent constipation.

Young children

Young children need to have plenty of foods containing protein for growth, and foods containing calcium and vitamin D to build up strong bones and teeth. (See chapter 16 for more on food for young children.)

Adolescents

Adolescents also need protein foods and calcium and vitamin D because they grow quickly at around age 11 for girls and 13–14 for boys. Girls especially should eat foods containing iron to replace that which is lost in menstruation.

The elderly

Elderly people need foods containing calcium and vitamin D because bones easily break as people become older. (Sunshine helps too.) Vitamin C from fresh fruit and vegetables will help prevent gum diseases.

Vegetarians

People who do not eat meat, eggs, milk or cheese for personal, religious or health reasons must plan their diets carefully. **Lacto vegetarians** do not eat meat, but they will eat milk, cheese and eggs, so they still get a good supply of protein. Strict vegetarians or **vegans** can only eat the protein contained in vegetable foods. They will need to eat a great variety of cereals, nuts and vegetables to get enough protein. Vitamin B12 is found mainly in animal foods so vegans may be short of this unless supplements are taken or foods to which B12 has been added are eaten. It is not as easy for the body to make use of iron from vegetables as it is from meat so vegetarians may need extra iron. (See chapter 8 for more on cooking for vegetarians.)

Invalids

People who are recovering from illness or injury need plenty of protein foods for repair of the body tissues, and vitamin C for healing wounds. All foods should be easy to digest. (See chapter 19 for more on cooking for invalids.)

Other things to consider

There are other things you should think about when planning meals.

Colour

An attractive choice of colours in a meal will make it seem more appetising and start the digestive juices working.

What do you think of this choice of foods?

Cod, cauliflower, creamed potatoes

Beetroot, tomato and carrot salad

How could you improve the choice of colour in these dishes?

Texture

All meals should contain some foods which are crunchy or need chewing. If all the food in a meal is soft, the food is easily swallowed without being chopped up and mixed with saliva to aid digestion.

How could you improve the texture in these meals?

Curried mince, rice
Ice cream

Steak and vegetable pie
Apple tart and custard

Flavour

Try not to repeat flavours, e.g. do not follow a fish starter with a fishy second course, or serve two courses with rice.

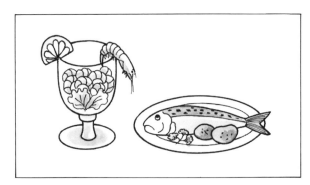

Figure 2.1

Do not forget to taste dishes before serving to make sure that the flavour is good and add other ingredients if necessary. Use herbs, spices and essences to develop flavours.

What would you serve as the other course with these meals?

Melon	Tomato soup
Chicken pie, carrots, peas	?
?	Fruit fool

Economy

Fuel

It is not economical to cook half the meal on the hob and the other half in the oven. This meal could be cooked entirely in the oven:

Moussaka (see recipe, page 63)
Conservative carrots (page 102)
Baked stuffed apples (page 118)

The automatic timer is useful when cooking meals such as this.

Think of a meal which could be made using only the hob and grill.

Using a pressure cooker or microwave cooker also saves fuel because cooking times are reduced.

For more about economy in the use of fuel see the section on energy saving in the book *Home and Consumer* in this series.

Money

Buy foods which are in season. Foods like avocado pears, strawberries and some vegetables are cheaper at certain times of the year.

Plan menus in advance so that you can arrange to use up left-overs in an economical way.

Buy in bulk where possible, e.g. dry goods, foods for the freezer.

Shop around for the best value — street markets are often cheaper for fruit and vegetables.

Time

Some people have less time for preparing and cooking food than others, e.g. parents who have a full time job and a family to bring up will probably not have much time for cooking an evening meal.

Labour saving equipment like mixers, liquidisers and food processors will help to

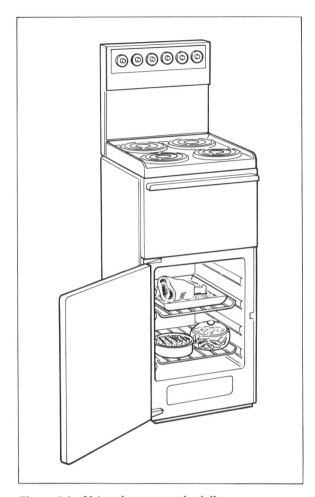

Figure 2.2 Using the oven to the full

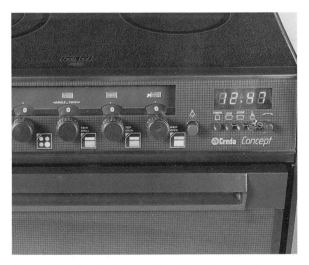

Figure 2.3 Controls for setting the automatic timer

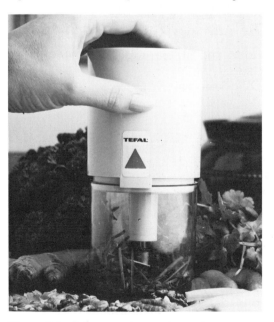

Figure 2.4 Labour saving equipment

speed up the making of a meal, and quick cooking methods like grilling or the use of a pressure cooker or microwave cooker will save time on cooking.

If your cooker has an automatic time control you can set it to turn on and off in your absence, but you will need to prepare dishes which can be left without spoiling (apples and potatoes would go brown unless part-cooked, and milk puddings can go rancid in hot weather if left in a gas oven with a pilot light).

Using **convenience foods** for all or part of a meal can also save time.

Convenience foods

These are foods that have been processed and packaged in such a way that they save time and effort.

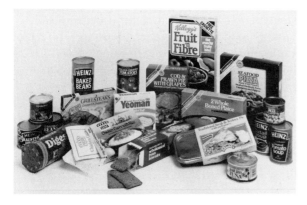

Figure 2.5   Some convenience foods

Unfortunately many convenience foods contain a large amount of fat, sugar and salt, so it is not a good idea to have them too often. They also tend to be expensive. Try always to read the label to see what you are actually buying. You may be surprised at all the extra ingredients or **additives** which have been put in to add flavour, colour or texture or to make the food last longer. These additives are sometimes just put in to make us buy the food and are not necessary in a healthy diet. We should try to avoid eating too many convenience foods containing additives.

The list of ingredients is always shown in

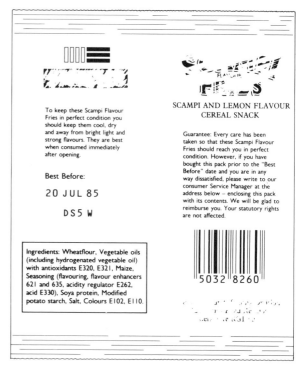

To keep these Scampi Flavour Fries in perfect condition you should keep them cool, dry and away from bright light and strong flavours. They are best when consumed immediately after opening.

Best Before:

20 JUL 85

DS5 W

SCAMPI AND LEMON FLAVOUR CEREAL SNACK

Guarantee: Every care has been taken so that these Scampi Flavour Fries should reach you in perfect condition. However, if you have bought this pack prior to the "Best Before" date and you are in any way dissatisfied, please write to our consumer Service Manager at the address below – enclosing this pack with its contents. We will be glad to reimburse you. Your statutory rights are not affected.

Ingredients: Wheatflour, Vegetable oils (including hydrogenated vegetable oil) with antioxidants E320, E321, Maize, Seasoning (flavouring, flavour enhancers 621 and 635, acidity regulator E262, acid E330), Soya protein, Modified potato starch, Salt, Colours E102, E110.

5032 8260

Figure 2.6   How many additives are there in this food?

order of quantities, *i.e.* with the ones there are most of at the top, so you can check whether you are buying more of the food or more of the additives. (See chapter 18 for more on convenience foods.) See the section on labelling in the book *Home and Consumer* in this series for work on food labelling.

Questions

1   Which of these meals would be the best choice nutritionally?

   (a)   Chicken with lemon and tarragon
   Jacket potatoes
   Hungarian beans
   Sponge flan

   (b)   Chicken Maryland (fried in
   breadcrumbs)
   Chips
   Strawberry cream gateau

Give reasons for your choice.

Table 2.1   Checklist for dishes

Dishes	Nutrition					Appearance/Taste				Cooking				
	High fibre (tick)	Low sugar (tick)	Low salt (tick)	Low fat (tick)	Variety of nutrients (list main ones)	Variety of colour (tick)	Variety of textures (tick)	Flavouring (list spices, herbs, etc.)	Presentation (list garnishes, decoration used)	Use of cooker (list parts used)	Equipment (list any equipment used, e.g. microwave cooker, food processor)	Cost	Time (used)	Practical skills (list practical skills used, e.g. preparing fruit/vegetables, making pastry)
Mediterranean peppers (see page 58)	✓	✓	✓	✓ (only if baked)	Fibre Protein Iron			Basil Tomato puree	Parsley	Top oven		M	P=15 C=40	Preparing vegetables
Brown rice	✓				Vitamin C Vitamin B1								C=40	
Hungarian beans (see page 101)	✓	✓	✓	✓	Vitamin B1 Vitamin C Fibre			Paprika		Top oven (or micro-wave)	Microwave cooker	C	P=10 C=15	Preparing vegetables
Melon salad with fruit, ginger & nuts (see page 43)		✓	✓	✓	Vitamin C			Ginger	Could use slice of lemon before squeezing			M	P=10	Preparing fruit
Strawberry Milkshake			✓	✓	calcium Vitamin D	✓	✓	Fruit	Nutmeg		Food processor	C	P=5	

E = Expensive
M = Medium
C = Cheap

P = Preparation time
C = Cooking time

2 In food examinations you will have to show that you understand the points made in this chapter and can put them into practice when choosing meals. You will be asked to make meals for people with different needs and for different occasions. You will be expected to work economically and show that you know some of the processes used in preparing food.

Make yourself a checklist like the one shown in the table on page 11 and tick off or fill in the sections for each dish.

This should help you to work out for yourself whether you have:

(a) shown a good knowledge of nutrition;
(b) made an economical choice of time, money and fuel;
(c) made suitable use of available equipment;
(d) chosen dishes which taste good and look attractive;
(e) shown that you are able to carry out the choice, preparation and serving of food.

The sample examination question below is answered in the table on page 11, which gives one possible set of dishes.

Sample question for a one-hour practical exam:
Current nutritional advice warns people against eating too much fat and sugar and encourages the use of more fruit and vegetables. Plan a day's meals for yourself and three friends which is based on the above advice. Prepare one of the day's meals and evaluate the outcome.

For more on eating during pregnancy, and on food for children, see *GCSE Home Economics: Families and Child Development*.

3 Methods of cooking

Why food is cooked

Food is cooked:

1 To destroy bacteria or to make them harmless.
2 To slow down unpleasant changes, e.g. apples would turn brown and go rotten if left uncooked.
3 To destroy natural poisons (toxins), e.g. red kidney beans must be boiled for at least 15 minutes to kill their toxins.
4 To make it more digestible.
5 To make it tender. Imagine chewing a hunk of raw meat.
6 To make it more appetising. Raw meat would not be very pleasant for example!
7 To improve flavour. Herbs, spices etc. can be added and these add flavour during cooking.
8 To add variety. Some foods can be cooked in different ways, e.g. beef can be roasted, made into a pie, casserole or mince dish.

Moist methods of cooking

Liquids, e.g. water, stock, are used.

1 Boiling (100°C)

Examples: rice, pasta, eggs.

2 Simmering (90°C)

Examples: meat, fish dishes, risotto, soup.

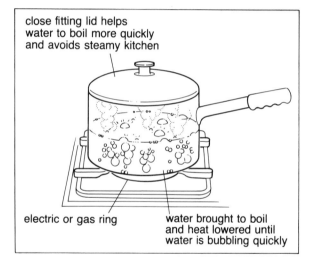

Figure 3.1 Boiling

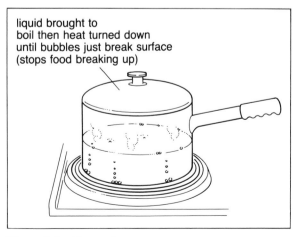

Figure 3.2 Simmering

3   Poaching

Examples: eggs, fish.

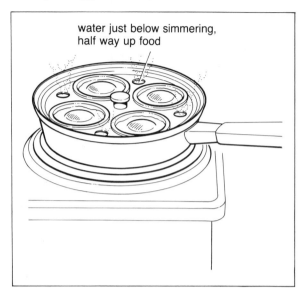

water just below simmering,
half way up food

Figure 3.3   Egg poacher

4   Par-boiling

This is part-cooking foods by boiling until the outside is just soft, then finishing off in a different way. For example, potatoes can be par-boiled before roasting. The par-boiling softens the outside of the food and cuts down cooking time. Potatoes end up with a crisp outside.

Nutrients can be lost into the water when boiling, simmering, steaming, poaching and par-boiling so use the liquid if possible, e.g. make it into gravy or a sauce.

5   Steaming

When foods are steamed they do not lose as many nutrients as in the other methods of moist cooking. The food is light and easy to digest and no fat is used, so dishes cooked in this way are good for invalids and for cutting down on fat. Steaming does take a long time and makes the air in the kitchen moist.
Examples: puddings, vegetables, meat, fish.

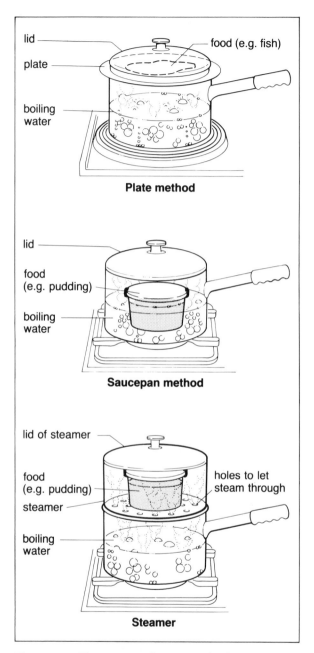

lid — food (e.g. fish)
plate
boiling water

Plate method

lid
food (e.g. pudding)
boiling water

Saucepan method

lid of steamer
food (e.g. pudding)
steamer
boiling water
holes to let steam through

Steamer

Figure 3.4   Three ways of steaming food

6   Pressure cooking

Water normally boils at 100°C. If the pressure inside the cooking pan is made greater the water will boil at a higher temperature. This is done by letting the air out and then stopping any steam

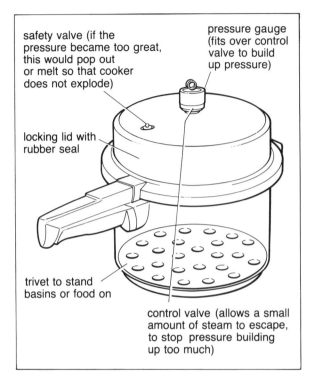

safety valve (if the pressure became too great, this would pop out or melt so that cooker does not explode)

pressure gauge (fits over control valve to build up pressure)

locking lid with rubber seal

trivet to stand basins or food on

control valve (allows a small amount of steam to escape, to stop pressure building up too much)

Figure 3.5   Pressure cooker

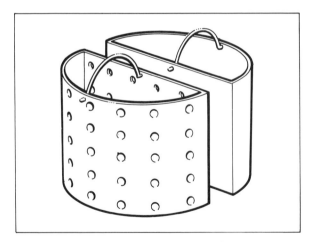

Figure 3.6   Separated containers to go in pressure cooker

from escaping with a special lid, with weights to set the pressure. Steam is forced through the food and it cooks very quickly. A meat dish will cook in 20 minutes instead of 2 hours.

Different foods can be cooked together in a separated container, saving fuel as well as time.

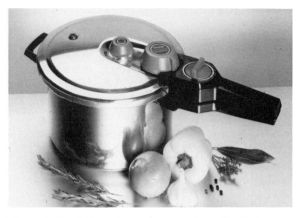

Figure 3.7   Automatic pressure cookers like this one have a timer to set and the steam is released automatically when the time is up. An alarm indicates that the heat should be turned off.

Examples: meat dishes, pulses, puddings, soup, jam, vegetables.

Fewer nutrients are lost because of the shorter cooking time, but some may be destroyed by the high temperature.

To use a pressure cooker

1   Put the food and liquid in the pressure cooker as it says in the recipe. N.B. Do not fill more than two-thirds full of liquid.
2   Make sure the rubber ring (gasket) is round the lid and not perished. Put the lid on and turn to seal.
3   Put the weights (pressure gauge) on as in the recipe. Put the pressure cooker on the top of the cooker on full heat.
4   Heat until there is a hiss from the pressure gauge. Turn the heat down until the hiss is gentle.
5   Heat for the time given in the recipe.
6   Lower the pressure by leaving the pan to stand off the heat *or* by standing the pan in a sink of cold water and running cold water over it (avoiding the safety valve and pressure gauge). Use oven gloves when handling the pressure cooker. To test whether the pressure is down, tip the weight slightly. If there is no steam the pressure has dropped and you can remove the lid.

7   Crockpot or slow cooker

A crockpot is an earthenware or stoneware pot with a metal or plastic case. There is a heating element under the base or around the sides of the pot. This heats to a very low temperature so food can be left for a long time to cook slowly to make it tender. Crockpots use very little electricity. Some foods like pulses and beans may not cook completely because of the low temperature. With red kidney beans this could be *dangerous* because they need to be boiled to kill off their poisons. Boil them for 15 minutes before adding to the crockpot. Because of the long slow cooking more vitamins may be destroyed in dishes cooked in this way. Example: casseroles of meat.

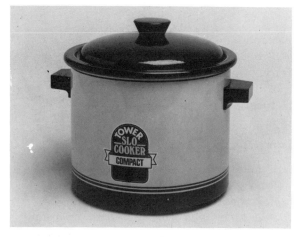

Figure 3.8   Slow cooker

8   Stewing

This is similar to boiling, but the food is cooked below boiling point. This can be done in the oven in a covered dish and it is then called casseroling. Stewing or casseroling makes food very tender and flavour develops. Washing-up is saved by cooking a whole meal in one dish. These dishes will need to cook for a long time. Examples: meat and vegetable dishes.

9   Braising

This is a mixture of roasting and stewing. Meat or fish is placed on a bed of vegetables (called a mirepoix) with just enough liquid to come up to the vegetables. The food cooks in the steam from the liquid. Meat cooked in this way is very tender, and it browns on the top as if it was roasted.
Examples: meat, poultry.

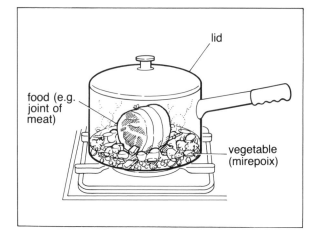

Figure 3.9   Braising

Dry methods of cooking

1   Pot-roasting

This is roasting which is carried out (on top of the cooker) in a heavy covered saucepan with a little fat.

2   Frying

This is cooking in fat or oil in a pan on top of the cooker. Too many fried foods are not good for us because of the amount of fat they contain. Use polyunsaturated vegetable oil rather than saturated fats like lard which has more cholesterol (see page 3). All fried foods should be well drained on kitchen paper to get rid of the extra fat.

Types of frying

1   *Shallow frying* — cooking with enough fat to cover the base of the pan.

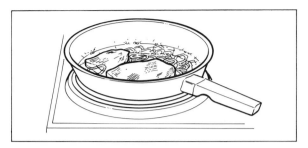

Figure 3.10   Shallow frying

Chinese stir frying uses a **wok** in which meat, fish and vegetables are cooked together, stirring constantly, in a little fat. The shape of the wok keeps the fat around the food.
Examples: tender cuts of meat, eggs, fish, vegetables.

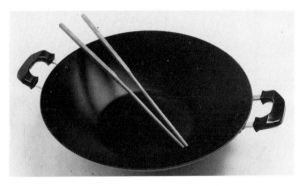

Figure 3.11   A wok

2   *Dry frying* — cooking in a very small amount of fat. This may be fat from the food which seeps out, e.g. bacon, or the pan may be greased.
Examples: chops, bacon.

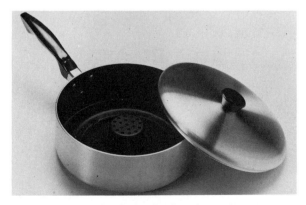

Figure 3.12   In dry fryers food cooks in the steam and is crispened by contact with the hot pan.

3   *Deep fat frying* — cooking food completely covered in fat.

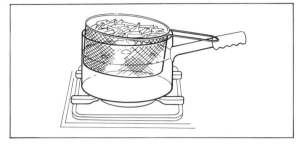

Figure 3.13   Chip pan and basket for deep fat frying

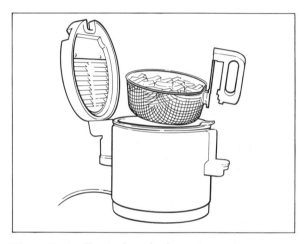

Figure 3.14   Elecric deep fat fryer

This can be done in a strong saucepan with a basket or in an electric fryer with a thermostat which turns the heat off when it reaches the set temperature.

Most foods need coating before deep fat frying:
(a)   to stop them breaking up;
(b)   to stop overcooking;
(c)   to help prevent the food soaking up too much fat.
Coatings could be:
    egg
    egg and breadcrumbs
    egg and flour
    egg and oatmeal
    batter
The egg in the coatings sets in the heat while the food inside cooks.
Examples: fish in batter, Scotch eggs, chips.

Some safety points for frying

Oil or fat reaches a very high temperature when it is heated. It can catch fire if overheated and cause very serious scalds if splashed or upset on the skin.

1   Do not overheat. The safest way to fry is to use a special thermometer. The fat should be at 150–195°C depending on the fat used and what is being cooked. Look up the correct temperature for what you are cooking.

    If you do not have a frying thermometer drop a small piece of bread into the fat or oil when you put it on to heat. When the bread floats to the top of the fat, bubbles and goes golden brown the fat is ready. It will go on heating up so turn the heat down once the food is bubbling gently.

    An electric deep fat fryer can be set to the correct temperature and it will keep turning itself on and off to keep the fat at the right temperature as the food cooks. It is much safer than frying on top of the cooker.

    The safest way, though, is *not to fry at all*, and it is better for your health.

2   Keep any pan used for frying at the back of the cooker with the handles turned inwards.

3   Never leave the room when frying without first turning off the heat. Do not leave children alone with fat pans.

4   Do not fill the pan more than two-thirds full of fat.

5   Keep a large lid or tin tray handy by the cooker when frying. If the fat catches fire turn the heat off and place the lid or tray on top of the pan, or throw a damp cloth over the pan.

6   Do not throw water on a burning fat pan or leave a kettle where it could splash into the fat. The hot fat will splash back at you.

3   Grilling

This dries the food up quickly, so sometimes oil or a moist sauce (baste) is spread on the food. This is a quick method of cooking and is good

for snacks. It allows the fat to drain out of foods which is good when trying to cut down on fats. Examples: thin cuts of meat, liver, kidney, fish fillets, tomatoes, mushrooms, toast.

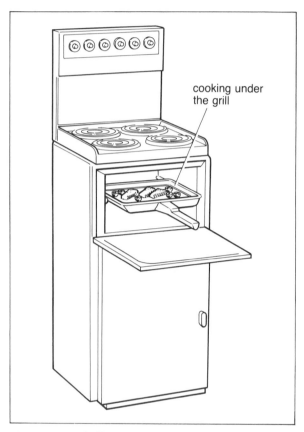

Figure 3.15   Grilling

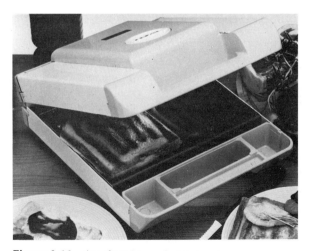

Figure 3.16   An electric sandwich toaster

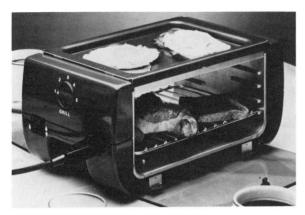

Figure 3.17 Table-top grills are useful for bed-sitters where there is no cooker.

4 Baking

Because hot air rises the top shelf in an oven is usually the hottest place. The middle and lower shelves may be 3–5°C cooler than the top shelf. Use the top shelf for things you want to go crisp like pastry and biscuits, the middle shelf for cakes and puddings and the bottom shelf for long slow cooking of things like casseroles. Some cookers have an electrically operated fan which helps to spread the heat more evenly in the oven.

Examples: jacket potatoes, cakes, biscuits, meringues.

5 Roasting

Examples: potatoes, chicken, meat.
It is usually possible to cook something else in the oven at the same time to save fuel.

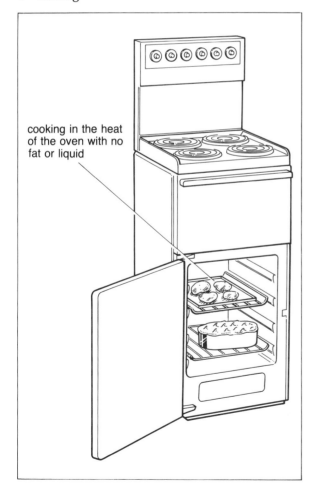

cooking in the heat of the oven with no fat or liquid

Figure 3.18 Baking

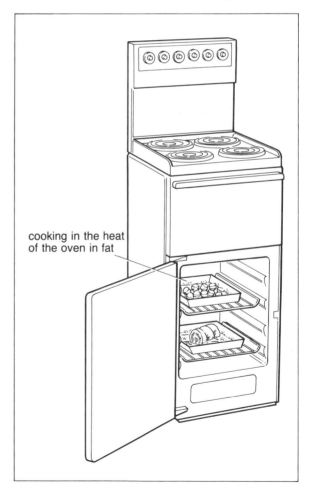

cooking in the heat of the oven in fat

Figure 3.19 Roasting

Microwave cooking

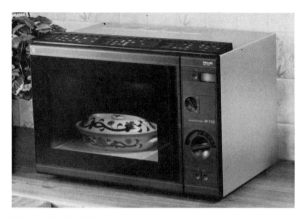

Figure 3.20   Microwave cooker

Energy can be transmitted in the form of electro-magnetic waves. This is known as radiation and is how light and heat from the sun reach the earth. If they are strong enough the waves can cause the temperature to rise in anything they touch and this is what microwaves do. Microwaves vibrate millions of times a second. If you rub your hands together the friction makes them warm; the microwaves do the same thing in food.

Containers for microwave cooking

Microwaves are reflected (bounced off) from metal, so metal containers cannot be used or the food would never get hot. (Some microwave cookers act like a normal cooker as well and metal can be used in these.)

Some materials let the microwaves through, but do not heat up themselves, e.g. paper, glass, china and plastics, so these make good containers for use in microwave cookers.

Some plastics scorch and give off unpleasant smells if used in the microwave, e.g. melamine, polystyrene, so avoid using containers made of these.

Advantages of a microwave cooker

1   Food cooks very quickly, e.g. a jacket potato will cook in 4–6 minutes instead of $1-1\frac{1}{2}$ hours.
2   The sides of the cooker and most dishes stay cool so the microwave cooker is useful for handicapped, elderly or young people.
3   Nutrients are not destroyed in the short cooking time, or lost in the liquid because only a little is needed.
4   Food does not burn on the inside of the cooker, so it is easy to clean.
5   The microwave plugs into a 13 amp socket so it is easily moved.

Disadvantages

1   Food does not brown, so it will need to be finished off under the grill or in the oven if a brown top is wanted.
2   It is easy to overcook food so check times carefully.
3   There are some cold spots in the microwave cooker — areas that are missed by the microwaves — which can lead to uneven cooking. It is necessary to turn the food occasionally to avoid this. Some models have a turntable or wave stirrer to cut down the likelihood of cold spots.

For more information about large and small equipment (cookers, freezers, refrigerators) and choosing equipment see *GCSE Home Economics: Home and Consumer*.

4 Understanding recipes

This chapter tells you things you may need to know to follow a recipe.

Food preparation

Halve
Put finger and thumb either side of knife for safety.

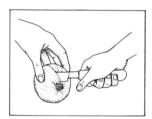

Quarter
With cut side down, cut in half again.

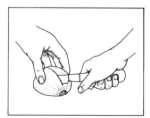

Chip
Cut in slices across the quarters.

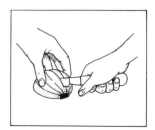

Dice
Cut in the other direction.

Chop
Cut in the other direction more closely.

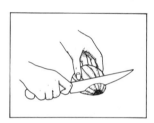

Chop finely
Hold pointed end of knife in place. Chop up and down, moving knife blade backwards and forwards.

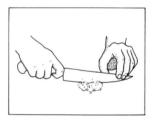

N.B. Fresh parsley or herbs can be quickly chopped by snipping with scissors into a cup or small basin.

Grate
Always grate downwards. The cutting edge is only in one direction, and you are less likely to grate your fingers.

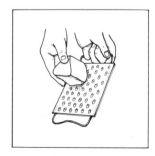

In a mouli grater the food is held still. Turning the handle moves the cutting edge round and this grates the food.

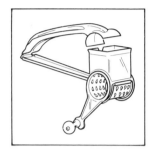

Garnishes

These are ways to decorate or to make food look attractive.

Tomato water lilies
Use a sharp pointed knife (with care) to make short zig-zag cuts through the tomato to the centre. Pull apart gently.

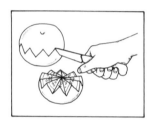

Cucumber twists (or lemon twists)
Cut thin slices of cucumber (or lemon). Cut across from one edge to the centre. Twist the ends in opposite directions.

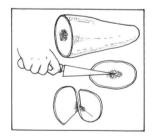

Celery curls
Cut sticks of washed celery into 8 cm lengths. Fringe each end with a sharp knife without cutting through the centre.
   Leave in ice cold water for at least half an hour until they curl.

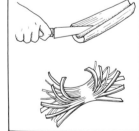

Bacon rolls
Flatten rashers of bacon with the back of a knife. Cut into 6–8 cm lengths. Roll up and thread on a skewer. Grill for 10 minutes, turning from time to time until cooked.

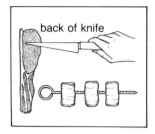

Gherkin fans
Slice gherkins lengthwise several times almost to the bottom. Spread out in a fan shape.

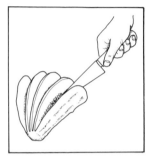

Lining tins

Lining tins helps to protect the food from burning and stops it sticking to the tin.

Cake tin
(a) Draw round the bottom of the cake tin on a sheet of greaseproof paper and cut out the circle.
(b) Cut a strip of greaseproof which is the height of tin + 5 cm, and long enough to reach round the tin. Make a fold along one edge 1.5 cm in. Snip the folded piece, diagonally, at 1 cm intervals.

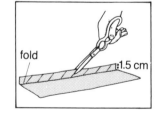

(c) Grease the tin by brushing with oil. Place the paper round the tin with the folded edge round the bottom.

(d) Place the circle in the bottom. Grease.

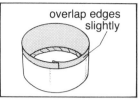

overlap edges slightly

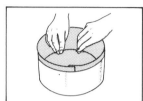

For large cakes which cook for a long time you may want to double-line tins for extra protection. Use two thicknesses of greaseproof paper and cut as above.

Swiss roll, or square, tin

(a) Draw round the bottom of the tin on a sheet of greaseproof paper which is the size of tin + depth + 2 cm.

(b) Fold the paper inwards on the lines you have drawn. Then unfold and cut diagonally from the corners of the paper to the corners of the square.

(c) Grease the tin. Place the paper in the tin with the folds around the bottom. Overlap the corners.

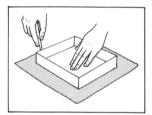

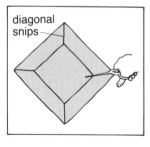

diagonal snips

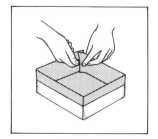

Conversion tables

g–oz conversions	
g (grams)	**oz (ounces)**
25	1
50	2
75	3
100	4
150	6
200	8 (i.e. $\frac{1}{2}$ lb)
225	9
250	10
300	12
400	16 (i.e. 1 lb)
800	32 (i.e. 2 lb)
1000 (1 kilogram)	2.2 lb

ml–pint conversions	
ml (millilitres)	**pints**
150	$\frac{1}{4}$
250	$\frac{1}{2}$
375	$\frac{3}{4}$
575	1
675	$1\frac{1}{4}$
800	$1\frac{1}{2}$
950	$1\frac{3}{4}$ (approximately 1 litre)

Note: all the conversions above are *approximate* to make the numbers rounded for easier use. Do not mix metric and imperial weights.

Oven temperatures		
Electricity °C	°F	Gas Reg (Mark)
100	225	$\frac{1}{4}$
120	250	$\frac{1}{2}$
140	275	1
150	300	2
170	325	3
180	350	4
190	375	5
200	400	6
220	425	7
230	450	8
240	475	9

About the recipes in this book

Flour

When the recipes call for 'wholemeal flour' or 'white flour' **plain** wholemeal or **plain** white flour should be used. When the recipes call for baking powder and white flour self-raising flour could be used instead.

Canned foods

Often the exact amount of canned food is not critical in a recipe. In these cases, the approximate can size is given (e.g. 'small can of baked beans', 'medium can of pears'). In other recipes that need more careful measurements the **weight** of canned food is given (e.g. '200 g of canned kidney beans').

5 Breakfasts

A healthy start to the day?

Each country has its own traditional breakfast; in England cereal, fried bacon, egg and bread, toast and marmalade, tea or coffee; in France coffee and croissants; in Holland bread, cold meats, cheese and chocolate; in India chapattis. The traditional English breakfast is high in fat and low in fibre and many people now try to make a more healthy start to the day by choosing from fresh fruit juice (no added sugar) or fresh fruit, and wholegrain cereal such as Weetabix, All-bran, muesli, or wholemeal bread and yogurt. These are quick to prepare and provides fibre and vitamins while cutting down on sugar and fatty foods. If a more filling breakfast is preferred, boiled or scrambled eggs may be eaten (but not too many times during the week as they are high in cholesterol), or lean meat or low fat cheese.

Why we need breakfast

Some people skip breakfast or just snatch a quick cup of coffee, and as a result start to feel tired, irritable or unable to concentrate by mid-morning. Breakfast literally means 'break fast' as it is the first meal the body has had for about eight hours. It is not very sensible to expect the body to cope with school or work for another three or four hours without fuel.

It is tempting when feelings of hunger do start to have a bar of chocolate or something else which is sweet. This makes you feel better for a while because it makes the level of sugar in the blood rise. The body then starts to produce insulin to deal with the extra sugar and the blood sugar level falls rapidly, leaving you feeling hungry again. It is better to eat foods which will help to keep the blood sugar level steady — nuts, seeds, raw vegetables, fruit, cheese or hard boiled eggs. So, eat a bag of nuts and raisins on the way to school if you have not got time for breakfast.

Questions

1 Think of some other ingredients you could add to breakfast muesli to ring the changes.

2 What other ingredients could be added to milk to make a nutritious breakfast drink?

3 Sometimes there is not enough time to cook for breakfast. What toppings could be quickly put together to go on crispbread or rolls?

4 Put these ideas together to form your own breakfast recipe leaflet.

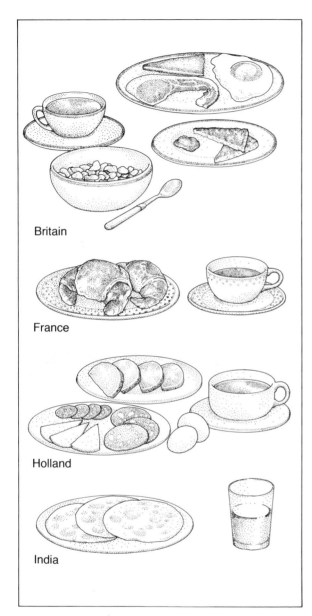

Britain

France

Holland

India

Figure 5.1   Breakfasts from around the world

Breakfast dishes

Some sample breakfast menus

Grapefruit
Welsh rarebit, toast, low fat spread, marmalade
Coffee

Fresh fruit juice
Scrambled eggs on toast
Wholemeal rolls, low fat spread, marmalade
Coffee

Stewed pears
Poached egg on toast
Bran muffins, low fat spread, apricot spread
Coffee

Grapefruit

Serve for breakfast, starter
Serves 2

Ingredients

1 grapefruit

Method

1   Scrub the outside of the fruit.
2   Cut the fruit in half horizontally. Remove the pips with the point of a knife.
3   Cut around each segment inside the pith. Serve in a glass dish.

If serving as a starter

Snip the peel in a zig-zag fashion. Place a half cherry in the middle.

Grilled grapefruit

Grapefruit may be served grilled, and hot, for a starter.

Ingredients

1 grapefruit
2 dessertspoons demerara sugar
1 teaspoon margarine

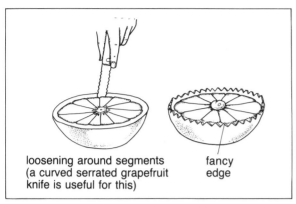

loosening around segments   fancy
(a curved serrated grapefruit   edge
knife is useful for this)

Figure 5.2

Method

1 Prepare as above.
2 Sprinkle with demerara sugar, dot with small pieces of margarine.
3 Grill until margarine has melted and top turns golden. Place cherry on top.

While it looks attractive, grilled grapefruit will, of course, have more kilocalories (kilojoules).

Fruit juice

Serve for breakfast, starter
Serves 1

Orange juice

Ingredients

1 orange

Method

1 Scrub the outside of the fruit.
2 Cut in half.
3 Squeeze out the juice using an orange squeezer.
4 Strain into a small glass.

Lemon juice (using liquidiser)

Ingredients

1 lemon
1 dessertspoon sugar
6 ice cubes

Method

1 Scrub the outside of the fruit.
2 Cut roughly into about 8 pieces.
3 Place in the liquidiser with the ice cubes.
4 Just cover with water. Add sugar.
5 Liquidise until the fruit is well broken up.
6 Strain into a glass.

Wake-up breakfast drink

Serve for breakfast, snack, for young children, invalids
Serves 1

Ingredients

1 pot natural yogurt
1 small orange
1 lemon
1 tablespoon honey

Method

1 Scrub the orange. Grate the rind finely.
2 Squeeze the juice from half the lemon.
3 Peel the orange. Break into segments and remove any pips.
4 Put the orange, lemon juice, orange rind, yogurt and honey into a liquidiser or food processor. Process until smooth.
5 Pour into a glass and serve.

Stewed (dried) fruit

Serve for breakfast
Serves 4

Ingredients

250 g whole fruit (e.g. prunes, figs)
or 150 g halved fruit (e.g. pears, peaches, apricots)
or 100 g sliced fruit (e.g. apple rings)
250 ml water
Lemon or orange rind, cinnamon stick or clove
Sugar to taste (omit if possible)

Method

1 Soak the fruit in the water with the flavourings overnight.
2 Pour into a saucepan. Bring to the boil, simmer for 20 minutes or until tender.
3 Add sugar to taste if necessary, but try to leave out.

or

Microwave method

1 Pour boiling water over fruit and flavourings. Microwave 1 minute. Leave to stand for 5 minutes.
2 Microwave 10 minutes or until tender.
3 Add sugar to taste if necessary, but try to leave out.

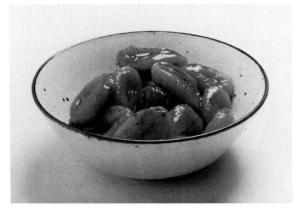

Figure 5.3   Bowl of stewed apricots

Muesli

Serve for breakfast
Serve with milk, yogurt, fresh fruit
Serves 4

Ingredients

75 g dried fruit (e.g. apricots, figs, dates, raisins, sultanas)
75 g nuts (e.g. almonds, hazelnuts, walnuts, cashews, peanuts)
100 g porridge oats
15 g sunflower seeds
1 pot natural yogurt *or* orange or apple juice (enough to moisten)

Method

1 Lightly toast the sunflower seeds under a hot grill.
2 Chop the fruit and nuts. This could be done in the food processor, but do not overdo.
3 Add the yogurt or fruit juice.
4 Soak overnight.
5 Add some fresh fruit if liked when serving.

Muesli makes a good 'between meals' snack, eaten dry, in place of something sweet.

Poached eggs

Serve for breakfast, snack
Serve with toast
Serves 1

Ingredients

1 egg
1 slice wholemeal bread
Low fat spread

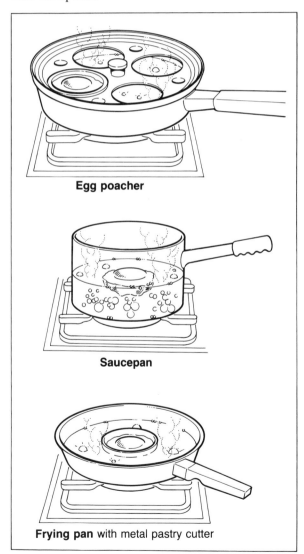

Egg poacher

Saucepan

Frying pan with metal pastry cutter

Figure 5.4   Three ways of poaching eggs

Method

Use an egg poacher, *or* a saucepan of fast boiling water, *or* a frying pan of water with a greased, metal pastry cutter in.
1   Bring the water to the boil.
2   Break the egg and drop gently into the poacher, water or pastry cutter. Cook until set.
3   Toast the bread. Spread with a little low fat spread.
5   Serve the egg on top of the hot toast.

The toast may be spread with Marmite before putting the eggs on. This will give extra vitamin B1 in addition to that in the wholemeal bread.

Scrambled eggs

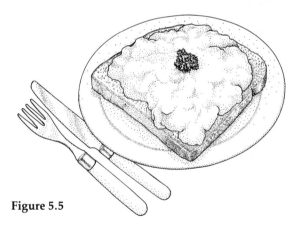

Figure 5.5

Serve for breakfast, snack
Serve with toast
Serves 2

Ingredients

3 eggs
2 slices wholemeal bread
Low fat spread
1 tablespoon skimmed milk
Small knob of margarine

Method

1 Break eggs into a small basin.
2 Add milk and whisk lightly with a fork.
3 Toast the bread lightly under the grill. Spread thinly with low fat spread. Place on serving plates and keep hot.
4 Place the knob of margarine in a saucepan. Melt over a low heat.
5 Add the eggs and stir gently with a wooden spoon until creamy.
6 Spread over the toast.

Microwave method

Scrambled eggs cook beautifully in the microwave oven, with no pan to wash.
1 Place the egg mixture in the basin in the microwave cooker. Cook 1 minute.
2 Stir. Cook further 35–50 seconds.

Additions

If serving for a snack you might like to add some grilled bacon or mushrooms or skinned tomatoes, chopped up and mixed into the egg mixture before cooking, or chopped parsley or chives mixed in just before serving. A sprig of parsley adds a splash of colour.

To skin tomatoes

Either place in boiling water and count to 20, pour off the water, cool and peel.
Or put on the end of a fork, hold in the gas flame, turning until the skin pops. Peel.

Welsh rarebit

Serve for breakfast, snack, starter
Serves 2

Ingredients

75 g firm low fat cheese
$\frac{1}{4}$ teaspoon mustard
2 tablespoons skimmed milk
2 slices wholemeal bread
Tomato
Parsley to garnish

Method

1 Make the toast. Keep hot.
2 Grate the cheese. Mix in the remaining ingredients to a paste.
3 Spread on the toast, covering well.
4 Brown lightly under the grill.
5 Skin and slice the tomato.
6 Arrange on the cheese and replace under the grill to warm through.
7 Garnish with a sprig of parsley.

As a starter

Omit the tomato above. Cut into small squares or triangles. Place a slice of tomato on each with a sprig of parsley in the middle.

Variation

For a more substantial dish try *Buck rarebit*. Make as for Welsh rarebit, but serve a poached egg on top.

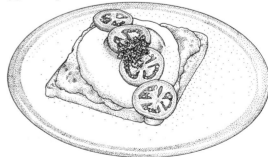

Figure 5.6   Buck rarebit

Bran muffins

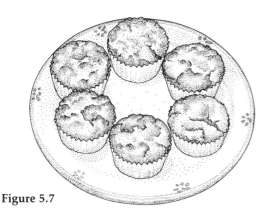

Figure 5.7

Serve for breakfast, tea, packed meal
Serve with low fat spread, marmalade or apricot spread
Makes 12

Cook at Reg 6
200°C
Time 25 minutes

Ingredients

100 g wholemeal flour
3 level teaspoons baking powder
50 g bran
1 level tablespoon caster sugar
1 orange
75 g dates, raisins, dried apricots or a mixture of all of these
1 egg
250 ml skimmed milk
25 g polyunsaturated margarine

Method

1. Put the oven on. Put paper cake cases in 12 bun tins.
2. Grate the rind of the orange finely.
3. Chop the fruit into small pieces.
4. Rub the margarine into the flour and baking powder.
5. Add the bran and sugar, the orange rind and the fruit.
6. Beat the egg lightly with the milk.
7. Add the milk and egg to the flour mixture and mix well with a fork.
8. Put teaspoons of the mixture into the bun tins.
9. Cook until golden brown and springy to touch.
10. Cool on a wire rack and serve warm or cold. They are best when fresh.

Bran muffins may be served in place of toast or rolls for breakfast. They are high in fibre and contain very little fat and sugar.

Apricot spread

Serve for breakfast, tea
Serve as a spread on breakfast muffins, wholemeal rolls
Makes 200 g

Ingredients

200 g dried apricots
1 tablespoon lemon juice
1 tablespoon thick honey (this may be left out)

This spread does not contain as much sugar as bought jams and marmalades. It also contains fibre.

Method

1. Soak the apricots in enough water to cover for a few hours *or* cover with boiling water and microwave for 1 minute, then leave to stand for 5 minutes.
2. Drain the apricots and chop finely.
3. Put the fruit in a liquidiser or food processor with the lemon juice and honey and blend until smooth.
4. Press into a clean, dry jam jar and eat within a week.

If you do not have a liquidiser or food processor you can cook the apricots to a purée with the lemon juice in a saucepan over gentle heat, or in the microwave. Then stir in the honey. Cooking must be very gentle to avoid burning.

6 Snack meals

There are times when we want a quick meal which is not the main meal of the day. It is very easy to snatch a bag of crisps, or a bar of chocolate, a doughnut or a bag of chips, or to buy convenience foods which do not take much time to cook.

But stop and think!

Is it fatty?

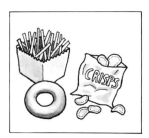

Is it high in sugar?

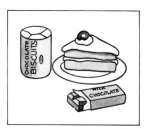

Is it salty?

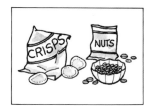

Is it full of additives?

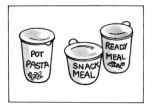

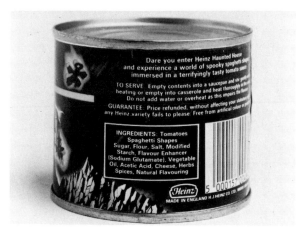

And do not forget the hidden sugar, salt and fat (or oil) in processed foods.

When you are buying a snack out you may not have a lot of choice, but if you are making something to eat at home you could choose food that is quick to prepare *and* provides some of the nutrients needed without being too fatty, salty and sugary.

Snack meals are not the same as *snacks* which are eaten *between* meals. If you really cannot wait until the next meal without something to nibble have some diced carrot, celery or cheese, unsalted nuts, dried fruits or dry muesli, rather than chocolate or biscuits.

Questions

1 Make a list of the foods eaten at 'breaktime' or at other times between meals by members of your class. Put them into groups under the headings:
high fat
high sugar
high salt
high fibre
low fat
low sugar
low salt

Make a poster, suitable for use with the youngest pupils at your school, to show how to eat healthily between meals.

2 Collect some labels from snack convenience foods, e.g. snackpots, frozen snacks.
List all the 'extra' ingredients you have when you buy processed foods. Many of these will be E numbers. These are ingredients added to change the flavour, texture or keeping properties of the food. Some people are ill if they have too many additives (see the chapter on 'Coping with Special Needs' page 166). Find out why these E numbers have been added (see *E for Additives**), and what side-effects they may cause.

Vegetable dishes

Tasty beans

Serve for snack
Serves 2

Ingredients

2 tablespoons water
1 small onion
Half a green pepper
175 g kidney beans — canned or cooked (see page 91)
Small can baked beans
2 tablespoons Worcestershire sauce
2 tablespoons tomato sauce
Shake black pepper
1 teaspoon mild chilli powder
75 g firm low fat cheese
2 slices wholemeal bread

Method

1 Put a serving plate to warm.
2 Peel and chop the onion.
3 Cut off the top of the green pepper. Remove the pith and seeds. Chop finely.
4 Drain the kidney beans.
5 Grate the cheese.
6 Cook the onion and pepper gently in water for 5 minutes until tender.
7 Add the kidney beans, baked beans, tomato sauce, Worcestershire sauce, pepper and chilli powder and stir well. Heat for 5 minutes.
8 Stir in the cheese and cook for 3 minutes or until the cheese has melted.
9 Toast the bread lightly on both sides.
10 Place the toast on the serving dish and pour the beans on top.

*Maurice Hanssen, *E for Additives*, Thorsons, 1984.

Surprise potatoes

Serve for snack,
accompaniment
Serve with salad or
baked beans
Serves 2

Cook at Reg 6
          200°C
Time 1–1½ hours
or Microwave 6–8 minutes

Ingredients

2 medium to large potatoes
Filling or topping (see below)

Surprise potatoes may have other ingredients
either mixed with the potato *or* as a topping.

Fillings

Cheese potatoes

50 g firm low fat cheese, grated (save a
    tablespoon of the cheese to sprinkle on the
    top of the potatoes)
3 drops of Worcestershire sauce
A little black pepper

Tuna and bacon potatoes

150 g tuna, flaked with a fork
50 g bacon, grilled and chopped

Toppings

Crispy bacon

75 g bacon, grilled, allowed to cool and
    crumbled

Mushrooms

50 g mushrooms, sliced and cooked gently in a
    little water until tender
1 tablespoon parsley, chopped

Onion

4–5 spring onions, chopped finely

Method

1   Put the oven on.
2   Scrub the potatoes well. Dry on kitchen
    paper or a clean teatowel.
3   Prick the potatoes with a fork.
4   Place on a baking tray and bake in the oven
    until tender. To microwave, place in a glass
    or china dish and cover with kitchen paper.
5   Test with a skewer or fork. The potatoes
    should feel soft.
6   While the potatoes are cooking prepare the
    filling or topping.
7   *For the fillings*   Cut the potatoes in half. With
    a teaspoon scoop out the inside of the
    potatoes into a bowl. Hold the potatoes in an
    oven glove as they will be hot, and try not to
    damage the skins. Mix the filling into the
    potatoes. Spoon the mixture back into the
    skins. For the cheese potatoes sprinkle a little
    cheese on top and grill until golden. For the
    tuna and bacon potatoes return to the oven
    for 15 minutes.
8   *For the toppings*   Make a crosswise slit on the
    top of each potato, and squeeze until the cut
    opens up. Put the chosen topping on and
    serve.

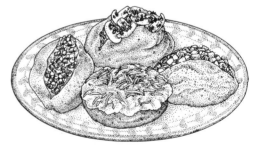

Figure 6.1

A microwave cooker really speeds up the time
for jacket potatoes:
        2 potatoes will cook in about 6–8 minutes
        3 potatoes will take about 9–11 minutes
        4 potatoes will take about 12–14 minutes
but this may vary a little depending on the type
of potato. The potatoes will need to stand for

about 10 minutes to soften after microwave cooking.

Egg dishes

See also Poached eggs (page 29)
Scrambled eggs (page 29)

Omelettes

Serve for snack
Serve with salad
Serves 1

Ingredients

2 eggs
2 tablespoons water
½ tablespoon vegetable oil
Parsley to garnish

Fillings

Any of these fillings can be put into the omelette mixture or folded inside the cooked omelette. Some fillings will need to be prepared before cooking the omelette.

1 teaspoon of parsley or other fresh herbs (chopped and added to the egg mixture)   *or*
30 g firm low fat cheese (grated and added to the egg mixture)   *or*
Lean chopped ham or grilled bacon   *or*
Mushrooms cooked in a little water until tender   *or*
Peeled, chopped tomato (see page 30 for peeling tomatoes)   *or*
Left-over cooked vegetables

Spanish omelette

Add chopped green and red peppers, onion, and cooked chopped potato to the omelette mixture before cooking. Do not fold this omelette, but serve flat.

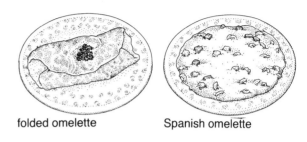

folded omelette   Spanish omelette

Figure 6.2   Two types of omelette

Method

1   Put a plate to warm.
2   Prepare any filling to be used.
3   Break the eggs into a basin. Add the water and whisk together with a fork. Stir in herbs, cheese or any of the fillings.
4   Heat the oil in a non-stick pan.
5   Pour the egg into the pan and keep it moving, stirring across the base of the pan. Tilt the pan to allow the uncooked mixture to run to the edges.
6   Allow to set and go golden on the bottom. If you are putting a filling inside, spoon this onto the omelette.
7   Fold one third over and fold again as you slide the omelette onto the plate.
8   Garnish with parsley.

Cheese dishes

Savoury supper dish

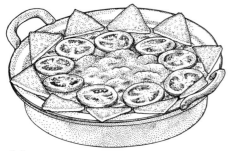

Figure 6.3

Serve for snack
Serve with toast
Serves 2

Ingredients

75 g firm low fat cheese
100 g lean ham
Small cauliflower
250 ml skimmed milk
1 tablespoon wholemeal flour
25 g polyunsaturated margarine
1–2 slices wholemeal bread
1 tomato

Method

1   Grate the cheese.
2   Cut the green leaves off the cauliflower.
    Break the cauliflower into small pieces.
    Cook in a saucepan of boiling water until
    tender (about 15 minutes) *or* microwave
    with 4 tablespoons of water for 12 minutes.
3   To make the sauce, place the margarine in a
    saucepan and melt gently. Add the flour
    and mix in with a wooden spoon. Cook
    gently for 1–2 minutes. Remove from the
    heat and stir in the milk adding only a few
    tablespoons at a time.
4   When all the milk is mixed in return the pan
    to the heat and bring to the boil stirring all
    the time with a wooden spoon. The sauce
    should thicken enough to coat the back of the
    spoon.
5   Add the grated cheese, saving a large
    tablespoonful for the top. Return the pan to
    the heat until the cheese just melts.
6   Toast the bread. Skin the tomato (see page
    30).
7   Drain the cauliflower and place in a
    heatproof serving dish. Chop the ham and
    sprinkle on top. Pour the sauce over the
    cauliflower.
8   Sprinkle the rest of the grated cheese over.
    Slice the tomato thinly and arrange on the
    top.
9   Brown lightly under the grill.
10 Cut the toast into triangles (these are called
    croûtons) and arrange round the edges.

This dish could also be made with wholemeal
pasta (e.g. macaroni or pasta shells) in place of
the cauliflower. This would provide more fibre
but no vitamin C. What could you have to follow
to provide this?

Hawaiian grill

Serve for snack
Serves 1

Ingredients

1 slice wholemeal bread
1 slice lean ham
30 g firm low fat cheese
1 pineapple ring
Small amount of low fat spread
Sprig of parsley, slice of tomato to garnish.

Method

1   Put a serving plate to warm.

2 Grate the cheese.
3 Toast the bread lightly on both sides.
4 Spread thinly with low fat spread.
5 Place the slice of ham on the toast.
6 Put the pineapple ring on the top.
7 Spread the grated cheese over. Grill until golden.
8 Garnish with sliced tomato and parsley and serve on the warm plate.

Fish and meat dishes

Crisp tuna casserole

Serve for snack, main meal
Serve with salad
Serves 3

Ingredients

25 g polyunsaturated margarine
25 g wholemeal flour
250 ml skimmed milk
Medium size can of tuna in brine
50 g wholemeal bread
75 g firm low fat cheese
A little black pepper
1 tomato

Method

1 Grease a 500 ml casserole dish.
2 Grate the cheese. Peel and thinly slice the tomato (see page 30).
3 Make breadcrumbs using the liquidiser, food processor or grater.
4 Drain off the brine from the tuna fish, and pat off the excess with kitchen paper. Flake with a fork.

5 Melt the margarine gently in a saucepan. Stir in the flour.
6 Remove from the heat. Stir in the milk *gradually*, about 2 tablespoons at a time.
7 When all the milk is added, return to the heat and bring to the boil stirring all the time with a wooden spoon. The sauce should be thick enough to coat the back of the spoon.
8 Stir in half the cheese, a shake of pepper and the tuna. Return to the heat until boiling again. Pour into the casserole dish.
9 Mix the remaining cheese with the breadcrumbs. Sprinkle over the top of the casserole.
10 Arrange tomato slices on top and grill until the top is golden.

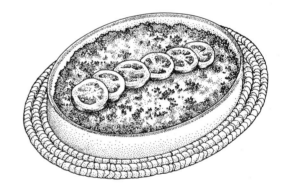

Figure 6.4

Risotto

Serve for snack, main meal
Serves 4

Ingredients

1 onion
50 g mushrooms
1 tablespoon vegetable oil
200 g brown rice
750 ml water + half a stock cube
Vegetables — *choose from:*
    stick celery
    red or green pepper
    a few peas or mixed vegetables
    tomato
Meat or fish — *choose from*:
    300 g liver
    300 g bacon
    medium size can of tuna in brine
    100 g prawns
    600 g cooked chicken
Parsley

Method

1   Put a serving dish to warm.
2   Prepare the vegetables. (Wash and chop the celery. Peel and chop tomatoes. Wash and slice mushrooms. Peel and chop onions. Wash and remove the seeds from peppers. Chop.)
3   If using tuna, drain and pat with kitchen paper.
4   Heat the oil in a large frying pan.
5   If using liver or bacon fry gently until cooked. Remove from the pan and chop into small pieces.
6   Add the onion to the pan. Fry gently until tender without browning.
7   Add the mushrooms and fry for a few minutes, then add the rice and heat together for 2–3 minutes.
8   Add the water and stock cube. Bring to the boil.
9   Add celery, peppers, tomato and simmer for 30 minutes.
10   Wash, dry and chop the parsley.
11   Add the rest of the vegetables and the meat or fish. Cook for 10 minutes more.
12   Serve on a large flat dish and sprinkle with parsley.

A risotto is a good way of using up left-over ingredients. You can have fun experimenting with different ingredients.

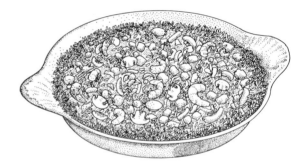

Figure 6.5

Hawaiian risotto

Add a small tin of pineapple, drained and chopped and 50 g raisins with the vegetables in bacon risotto. Garnish with sliced hard boiled eggs.

Colourful risotto

Add ¼ teaspoon turmeric.

7 Starters

This chapter is about **starters** — the first course of a meal. The correct name for a starter is an 'hors-d'oeuvre' which is French for 'outside the main work'. Traditionally it was small portions of food to get the digestive juices working and give people an appetite.

Starters are often served as the first course of a three course meal when entertaining, but most of us have simpler meals for every day. There is no reason, though, why you should not have a starter instead of a sweet for a two course meal. It will probably help in cutting down sugar and fats.

There are six different types of starter you can have:

Soups
Fruit/vegetable
Pâté/dips
Fish
Egg
Cheese

Soups

Soups are made from meat, fish or vegetables cooked in water with flavourings, called stock. Soups help digestion by getting the gastric juices going, and hot soups are satisfying in cold weather. You can provide extra nutrients by serving with, for example, wholemeal rolls or cheese.

Types of soup

1 Clear soup or consommé: a very thin, clear soup, usually served with a garnish of strips of vegetables.
2 Broth: clear soup with small pieces of meat, rice, oats or pasta, e.g. Scotch broth.
3 Thickened or cream soups: these are soups which are thickened with cornflour, flour, beaten egg or cream just before serving, e.g. cream of tomato soup.
4 Purées: these are very thick soups in which the ingredients are sieved or liquidised. Sometimes they are thickened with flour or cornflour as well, e.g. lentil soup.

Stock

Stock is a well flavoured liquid which is used to make soup. It can be made by dissolving stock cubes in water. Stock cubes are convenient to store in the cupboard and have handy when you need them, but they are very high in salt and fat. Use half a stock cube rather than a whole one to cut down on salt and do not add any other salt.

Stock can also be made by boiling up vegetables (but not green vegetables which can taste bitter) or bones from meat, fish or poultry, and giblets. The water left over from cooking vegetables makes a good stock as it contains the vitamins which would otherwise be washed down the sink. Do not use fatty parts of meat or you will have a greasy stock.

To make your own stock

1 Place vegetables, meat or fish bones in a large deep saucepan.
2 Just cover with water.
3 Add a bouquet garni. This is a small bag of herbs which will add flavour. Bouquet garni can be bought, but it is cheaper to make your own. Put 2–3 parsley sprigs, a pinch of thyme and a bayleaf into a piece of muslin and tie with string. This can be fished out when the stock is ready. Cover with a tight-fitting lid.
4 For meat or vegetable stock simmer for 2–3 hours. You can use a pressure cooker and then this will only take 40–60 minutes.
   For fish stock simmer for 45 minutes or pressure cook for 5 minutes.
   Stock can also be made more quickly in the microwave cooker, but it is not as tasty.
5 Strain into a jug, cool and then put in the refrigerator until ready for use. Any fat should set on the surface and can be removed before using the stock.
Stock can be frozen in margarine tubs or plastic pots so you always have some at hand.

Questions

1 Plan four two-course meals in which a starter is used instead of a sweet. One should be suitable for a low fat diet, one for a high fibre diet and one for a person who is slimming.
2 Find some recipes for other types of soup. List the ones which are high in fibre.
3 Invent another recipe for a fruit starter. List the nutrients it will provide.

Serving soup

1 Allow 150 ml of soup per person.
2 Soup can be served with:
   (a) croûtons (wholemeal bread toasted and cut into small squares);
   (b) grated cheese (e.g. parmesan cheese with minestrone soup);
   (c) chopped parsley;
   (d) strips of carrot or celery;
   (e) wholemeal rolls.

Cream of sweetcorn soup

Serve for starter
Serve with croûtons
Serves 4

Ingredients

Medium sized can sweetcorn
2 medium sized potatoes
1 onion
1 tablespoon vegetable oil
1 rounded tablespoon wholemeal flour
500 ml skimmed milk
250 ml water
1 bayleaf
Pinch black pepper
Parsley

Method

1 Peel and slice the potatoes and onion finely.
2 Heat the oil in a saucepan. Add the potato and onion and cook gently together until soft, but not coloured.
3 Wash, dry and chop the parsley.
4 Stir the flour into the potato and onion mixture.
5 Gradually stir in the milk and water.
6 Add the bayleaf and pepper.
7 Simmer gently for 15–20 minutes. Allow to cool slightly.
8 Liquidise or food process (or sieve) the soup.
9 Reheat and serve in soup bowls sprinkled with parsley.

Leek and potato soup

Serve for starter
Serve with croûtons, parsley
Serves 4

Ingredients

200 g potatoes
200 g leeks
1 onion
Shake of black pepper
300 ml water + half a chicken stock cube
200 ml skimmed milk
2–3 sprigs of parsley
2 slices wholemeal bread

Method

1   Wash and peel the potatoes. Cut into small
    pieces. Wash and slice the leeks.
2   Peel and slice the onion.
3   Put the onion, leeks, potatoes in a saucepan
    with the water and stock cube. Simmer for 30
    minutes or until the vegetables are tender.
4   Wash, dry and chop the parsley finely.
5   Toast the bread and cut into small cubes.
6   Place the soup in the liquidiser and liquidise
    for 1 minute or press through a sieve with a
    wooden spoon.
7   Return the soup to the pan. Add milk and
    pepper. Reheat, but do not boil. Serve in
    soup bowls and sprinkle with parsley. Serve
    the croûtons separately in a small bowl.

Lentil soup

Serve for starter
Serve with croûtons
Serves 4

Ingredients

1 onion
1 carrot
150 g lentils
500 ml water + half a chicken stock cube
1 bayleaf
250 ml skimmed milk
2 teaspoons lemon juice
Shake of black pepper
2 slices wholemeal bread

Method

1   Peel and chop the onion.
2   Peel and slice the carrot.
3   Wash and drain the lentils.
4   Place the onion, carrot and lentils in a
     saucepan with the bayleaf, stock cube and
     water.
5   Bring to the boil, then simmer for 30
     minutes or until the vegetables are tender.
6   Toast the bread and cut into small cubes.
7   Pour the soup into a liquidiser and liquidise
     for 1 minute or press through a sieve with a
     wooden spoon.
8   Add milk, lemon juice and pepper.
9   Reheat soup gently but do not let it boil.
10   Serve soup in a large soup bowl and
     croûtons in a small bowl.

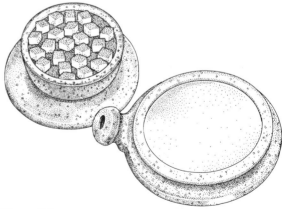

Figure 7.1

Watercress soup

Serve for starter
Serve with croûtons
Serves 4

Ingredients

2 bunches watercress
1 tablespoon vegetable oil
500 ml water + half a chicken stock cube
2 egg yolks
150 ml natural yogurt
Pinch black pepper

Method

1   Wash the watercress. Remove some of the leaves and save for a garnish.
2   Chop the rest of the watercress.
3   Peel and chop the onion.
4   Put the watercress, stock, onion, and pepper in a saucepan and bring to the boil.
5   Turn the heat down and simmer for 20 minutes. Cool slightly.
6   Food process or liquidise (or sieve) the soup.
7   Mix the egg yolks and yogurt together.
8   Stir a little of the soup into the yogurt mixture.
9   Return the soup to the rinsed out saucepan. Mix in the yogurt mixture.
10 Heat through without boiling.
11 Pour into bowls and garnish with watercress leaves.

Cucumber, lemon and mint soup (a chilled soup)

Serve for starter
Serve with wholemeal rolls
Serves 4

Ingredients

1 onion
Half a cucumber
1 tablespoon vegetable oil
450 ml natural yogurt
300 ml water + half a chicken stock cube
1 lemon
8 sprigs of mint
Black pepper

Method

1   Wash the mint. Save some leaves for decoration. Chop 2 tablespoons mint.
2   Peel and finely chop the onion.
3   Wash and grate the rind of the lemon. Squeeze out the juice.
4   Peel the cucumber and cut into 5 mm slices.
5   Heat the oil in a saucepan. Cook the onion gently for 3 minutes. Add the cucumber and cook for 5 more minutes.
6   Turn the vegetables into a bowl and leave to cool.
7   Dissolve the stock cube in a small amount of boiling water. Make up to 300 ml with cold water.
8   Stir the yogurt and stock into the cucumber mixture with the lemon rind and juice, mint and pepper.
9   Chill in the refrigerator for 1 hour.
10 Pour into individual bowls and garnish with sprigs of mint. Serve chilled.

Fruit starters

Fruit starters are usually citrus fruits or melon — light dishes which are not too filling. They add extra vitamin C and make a colourful and pleasant start to a meal without adding too many kilocalories (kilojoules).

See Grapefruit (page 26)

Melon boats

Serve for starter, sweet
Serves 3

Ingredients

Half a small melon
1 orange
3 cherries
3 cocktail sticks

Method

1 Scrape the pips from the centre of the melon. Cut the melon into three pieces.
2 Loosen the melon from the skin by slicing with a knife between the skin and the fruit, being careful not to cut the skin, or your hand.

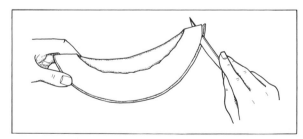

Figure 7.2 Cutting melon from skin

3 Cut in 1½ cm slices across the melon.
4 Arrange the slices sticking out on alternate sides of the melon.
5 Scrub the orange. Keeping the skin on, cut into thin slices.

6 Put the cocktail stick through the orange slice and press into the middle of the melon. Place a cherry on top.

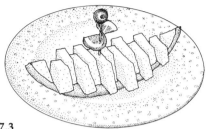

Figure 7.3

7 Serve on a shallow dish or saucer. A little powdered ginger may be served with the melon, sprinkle on top, if liked.

Melon salad with fruit, ginger and nuts

Serve for starter, sweet
Serves 4

Ingredients

2 oranges
1 lemon
25 g sultanas
25 g whole hazelnuts
½ teaspoon ground ginger
Half a melon

Method

1 Squeeze the juice from 1 orange and the lemon.
2 Put the sultanas and ginger in the juice to soak.
3 Peel the skin from the second orange and cut into segments.
4 Remove the skin and seeds from the melon. Chop.
5 Mix the melon, nuts and orange with the juice.
6 Spoon into small bowls.

Avocado, orange and nut cocktail

See colour photo (page 60)

Serve for starter
Serves 4

Ingredients

2 avocado pears
2 oranges
30 g nuts, e.g. walnuts, almonds, hazelnuts
Powdered nutmeg

Method

1 Halve the avocado pears. Scoop out the flesh. Chop into small pieces.
2 Peel and segment the oranges (see Figure 7.4). Cut the segments into smaller pieces.
3 Break the nuts into small pieces (not too small).
4 Mix the avocado, orange and nuts together.
5 Heap the fruit and nut mixture back into the avocado shells. Sprinkle a little powdered nutmeg on top.
6 Serve on a small dish.

Gold and silver cocktail

Serve for starter, sweet
Serves 3

Ingredients

2 oranges
2 grapefruit
2 cherries
Egg white and a little caster sugar to decorate
    the edge of the dish

Method

1 *To decorate the edge of glass dishes*   Whisk the white of egg lightly. Put the egg white on one shallow plate, the caster sugar on another. Dip the rims of the dishes alternately in the egg white, then the sugar. When dry they will sparkle.
2 Cut the rind from the fruit making sure you cut the pith off.

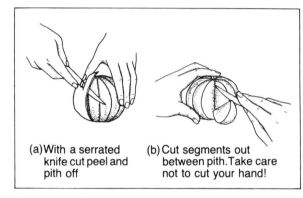

(a) With a serrated knife cut peel and pith off   (b) Cut segments out between pith. Take care not to cut your hand!

Figure 7.4   Preparing the fruit

3 Cut out the segments over a plate to catch the juice.
4 Arrange the slices alternately in the dishes. Chop any left-over slices and place in the middle.
5 Pour the juice over.
6 Decorate with half a cherry.

Pâté/dips

Pâté is a paste made from meat, liver or vegetables flavoured with herbs. Some pâtés are high in fat. Dips are softer and usually made from vegetables or cheese. Pâté is generally served with toast, and dips with strips of fresh vegetables (crudités) which can be dipped in (see colour photo, page 60).

Smoked mackerel pâté

Serve for starter
Serve with toast, salad
Serves 4

Ingredients

200 g smoked mackerel fillets
125 g cottage cheese
150 ml natural yogurt
Pinch of nutmeg and cayenne pepper
50 g polyunsaturated margarine
Parsley
1 lemon

Method

1 Cut the lemon in half and squeeze the juice
   from one half.
2 Scrape the skin from the fish and remove any
   small, loose bones.
3 Put the fish, cheese, yogurt, nutmeg, pepper,
   margarine and 1½ tablespoons lemon juice
   into a liquidiser or food processor. Process
   until well broken up, or until very smooth if
   a smoother pâté is liked.
4 Pour into individual dishes or one large dish.
5 Put into the refrigerator and leave to set.
6 Garnish with chopped parsley and lemon
   slices or butterflies.

Lemon butterflies
Lemon slices can be made into butterflies to
garnish dishes. Cut the lemon slices in half.
Cut in quarters almost to the centre and
arrange on top of the pâté.

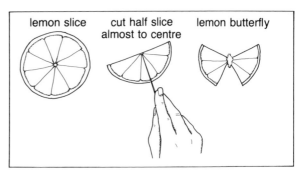

Figure 7.5 Making lemon butterflies

Hummus

See colour photo (page 60)

Serve for starter, buffet
Serve with fresh vegetable strips, toast
Serves 4

Ingredients

225 g cooked (see page 90) or canned chickpeas
1 small onion
2–3 tablespoons tahini (sesame seed paste)
Juice of 1 lemon
2 tablespoons vegetable oil
Sprigs of mint or black olives to garnish
Bread for toasting *or* fresh vegetables, e.g.
   carrot, celery, spring onion, to serve as an
   accompaniment

Method

1 Peel the onion and cut into quarters.
2 Make the chickpeas and onion into a purée in
   a liquidiser or food processor.
3 Add the tahini, lemon juice and oil and mix
   to a smooth purée. If it seems too thick add
   some of the juice from cooking the chickpeas.
4 Pile into a shallow serving dish and garnish
   with sprigs of mint or olives.
5 Serve with fingers of toast, *or* with strips of
   fresh vegetables (crudités) which can be
   dipped in.

Fava (Brown bean salad)

Serve for starter, buffet
Serve with toast, salad, strips of fresh vegetables
Serves 4

Ingredients

250 g cooked fava beans or any brown beans
    (see page 90)
1 large onion
Juice of 1 lemon
2 tablespoons vegetable oil
1 tablespoon natural yogurt
1 teaspoon dried dill
Parsley
Bread for toasting *or* fresh vegetables, e.g.
    celery, carrot, spring onion, to serve as an
    accompaniment

Method

1 Wash and chop the parsley.
2 Put the beans, lemon juice, oil, yogurt and
   dill in the food processor or liquidiser.
3 Process until smooth.
4 Pile in a shallow dish.
5 Sprinkle chopped parsley over.
6 Serve with fingers of toast or strips of fresh
   vegetables.

Egg and cheese starters

Egg mayonnaise

Hard boiled eggs may be coated with
mayonnaise and served on a bed of lettuce.
Sprinkle with cayenne pepper for a splash of
colour.

Devilled eggs

Serve for starter
Serve with lettuce
Serves 4

Ingredients

4 eggs
$\frac{1}{2}$ tablespoon mayonnaise
1 teaspoon curry powder
Lettuce
Cayenne pepper

Method

1 Wash, drain and dry the lettuce.
2 Hard boil the eggs. Cool in cold water. Slice
   lengthwise.
3 Remove yolks with a teaspoon handle.
4 Press the yolks through a sieve with a
   wooden spoon into a small basin.
5 Add the mayonnaise and curry powder.
6 Spoon or pipe the mixture back into the egg
   whites.
7 Place lettuce leaves on a serving dish with
   the eggs on top. Sprinkle with cayenne
   pepper.

Cheese starters

See Welsh rarebit (page 30).

Fish starters

Shellfish such as prawns make a more expensive starter. They are very salty so should be served with a meal which does not have many other salty foods.

Prawn cocktail

Serve as starter
Serve with lettuce, tomato, lemon
Serves 4

Ingredients

150 g peeled prawns
1 tablespoon mayonnaise
$\frac{1}{2}$ teaspoon tomato purée
Lettuce
Half a lemon
Cayenne pepper
1 tomato

Method

1 Wash the lettuce. Drain and dry on kitchen paper.
2 Scrub the lemon. Cut into quarters.
3 Mix the mayonnaise with the tomato purée. Gently stir in the prawns.
4 Shred the lettuce by tearing apart. Wash and slice the tomato.
5 Place a little lettuce in the bottom of each serving dish.
6 Place the prawn mixture on the lettuce.
7 Sprinkle with a little cayenne pepper.
8 Serve with a wedge of lemon and sliced tomato.

Avocado, grapefuit and prawn cocktail

Serve as starter
Serve with lettuce and lemon wedges
Serves 4

Ingredients

2 avocado pears
1 grapefruit
75 g peeled prawns
Lettuce
Half a lemon

Method

1 Wash the lettuce. Drain and dry on kitchen paper.
2 Scrub the lemon. Cut into quarters.
3 Halve the avocados. Scoop out the flesh and chop.
4 Slice the peel from the grapefruit and cut into segments (see page 44). Cut into smaller pieces.
5 Mix the grapefruit, avocado and prawns together.
6 Shred the lettuce by tearing apart.
7 Place a little lettuce in the bottom of each serving dish.
8 Place the avocado shells on the lettuce and fill with the prawn mixture.
9 Serve with a wedge of lemon.

8 Main meals

The main meal of the day, whether it is eaten at midday or in the evening, will need to provide a large amount of the nutrients needed by the body each day. It is important to include some protein in the form of meat, poultry, fish, cheese, eggs, pulse vegetables or nuts.

Meat dishes

Meat

Most meat is quite fatty. Not only does it have the fat you can see on the outside, but it also contains fat inside that you cannot see. Red meat contains more fat than white, so it is a good idea to cut down on red meat and to choose lean cuts. Eating more chicken or white fish also helps to cut down on fat. You can also try mixing vegetables like pulses with meat. This will be cheaper as you need less meat and will also add fibre as well as cutting down on fat. The fattiest meats are sausages, luncheon meat, salami, liver sausage and pork pies (fatty pastry as well as meat). Mince needs to be chosen with care. You can usually see lumps of fat in cheaper mince, but for only a little more money you can often buy a good quality mince.

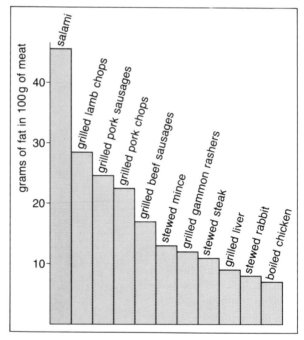

Figure 8.1 The amount of fat in different kinds of meat. Which two meats contain the least fat?

Meat, especially offal (see below), also provides iron as well as protein and pork provides vitamin B1.

The main meats eaten in the UK are:
    beef
    veal (calf)
    lamb (mutton is old lamb)
    pork (also as bacon)
    rabbit
We also eat:
(a)   **offal** — the internal organs of the animal,
       e.g. liver, kidneys, tripe, heart (offal is high
       in cholesterol, although fairly low in fat);
(b)   **poultry** — chicken, turkey and duck.

Cooking meat

Meat is cooked:

(a) To make it easier to eat and digest
Meat is the muscle of the animal and some
parts will be tougher than others depending on
where it comes from in the animal, e.g. the leg
will be well worked and therefore tougher. The
muscle fibres are held together with *connective
tissue* and during cooking this tissue softens and
makes the meat easier to eat.

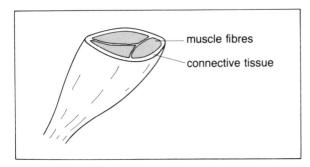

Figure 8.2   Muscle fibres in meat

In general tougher cuts of meat are cheaper
and need longer, slower moist cooking such as
stewing, casseroling, boiling. The more
expensive tender cuts can be roasted, grilled,
fried or braised.

(b) To make it safe to eat
Food poisoning can be caused by eating meat
which is not fresh.
1   Always buy meat which looks moist and has
     a good colour, and which does not have
     yellowing fat.

2   Cook the meat as soon as possible and do not
     leave it anywhere warm. Put it in the
     refrigerator until ready to use, and do not let
     meat juices drip onto other foods.
3   Never partly cook meat and reheat the next
     day. Germs multiply in warm conditions and
     when meat is only partly cooked the inside of
     the joint is only warm and not hot enough to
     kill germs. Cook the meat right through, cool
     it quickly and store in the refrigerator.
4   Be especially careful with pork, and chicken.
        Undercooked pork can give you *tapeworms*
     which will live in your intestines, feed off
     your food and make you very ill.
        All chickens contain *Salmonella* bacteria.
     These must be killed by cooking the chicken
     thoroughly or you may suffer from
     salmonella poisoning which is very
     unpleasant and can kill. These bacteria will
     get onto your hands when you handle the
     chicken (especially the inside of the chicken)
     and onto work surfaces, knives and dishes. It
     is important to wash everything which comes
     into contact with the chicken in mild bleach
     (half an egg-cup in a gallon of water). Be very
     careful that uncooked chicken does not come
     into contact with other foods in the
     refrigerator. If you have a frozen chicken it
     will need to be thawed completely before
     cooking otherwise some parts of the chicken
     may look cooked while other parts in the
     centre are still raw. Do not refreeze once you
     have started to thaw the chicken.

(c) To make it taste and look better

Questions

1   One way to cut down on fat in the diet
     would be to have one or two meatless days
     every week. Plan 3 days' meals which do not
     include the use of meat.
2   Plan a day's meals for someone recovering
     from a heart attack. What advice would you
     give about a diet to help prevent heart
     disease?
3   The numbers of deaths from diseases related
     to food are different in different countries.
     Find out about the type of food eaten in

Greece, Japan, Italy and Norway. In which countries is the type of food eaten most likely to increase the chance of heart disease or strokes?

4   Cheese can be very high in fat unless it is a low fat variety. Invent two toppings for a pizza which do not use cheese.

5   Make a list of the flavourings which have been used in dishes in this recipe book instead of salt.

The meat recipes

These are arranged in order with the meat containing least fat first. There are several recipes for each type of meat.

Chicken and ham loaf

Serve for main meal
Serve with potatoes,
a fresh vegetable and
tomato sauce (see page
113), or with salad
Serves 4

Cook at Reg 6
      200°C
Time 30–40 minutes

Ingredients

200 g cooked chicken
200 g cooked ham
75 g wholemeal bread
2 large sprigs of parsley
1 level teaspoon powdered mustard
2 eggs

N.B. In recipes where *cooked* chicken is needed, cook the chicken by (a) roasting in the oven for 20 minutes per 400 g + 20 minutes, *or* (b) pressure cook in enough water to cover for 7 minutes per 400 g, *or* (c) microwave, covered, for 8 minutes per 400 g.

Method

1   Put the oven on.
2   Grease and line the bottom of a 400 g loaf tin and grease a piece of greaseproof paper large enough to cover the top.
3   Mince the chicken, ham and bread. You could use the food processor for this.
4   Mix all the ingredients together.
5   Spoon into the loaf tin, pressing well into the corners.
6   Bake covered with greaseproof for 30–40 minutes.
7   Allow to cool for a few minutes.
8   Turn out onto a plate.
9   Serve with tomato sauce poured round or with salad arranged round the bottom.

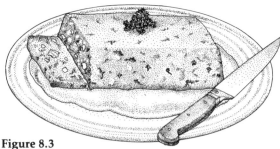

Figure 8.3

Chicken fricassée

Serve for main meal, for invalids
Serve with fresh vegetables
Serves 3

Ingredients

200 g cooked chicken
25 g wholemeal flour
25 g polyunsaturated margarine
250 ml skimmed milk
2 teaspoons lemon juice
Few sprigs of parsley
50 g bacon
400 g potatoes + a little skimmed milk
Small can sweetcorn

For a change add some cooked mushrooms to the sauce.

Method

1   Scrub, peel and boil potatoes until tender (about 20 minutes).
2   Mash and sieve.
3   Pipe around the edges of a shallow serving dish.
4   Chop parsley.
5   Bone and chop chicken.
6   Flatten the bacon by scraping flat with a knife, and roll up.
7   Melt the margarine in a non-stick saucepan. Stir in the flour. Remove from the heat.
8   Add the milk gradually, stirring in with a wooden spoon.
9   Return to the heat and bring to the boil stirring all the time with a wooden spoon.
10 Stir in the chicken and parsley. Add a little pepper if liked and the lemon juice.
11 Pour into the middle of the potato.
12 Grill the bacon rolls and use to garnish the top.
13 Heat the sweetcorn. Drain and arrange round the edges of the potato.

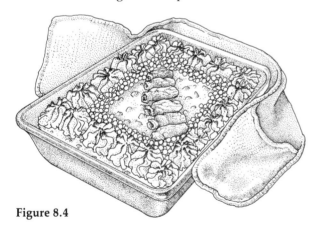

Figure 8.4

Spicy chicken

See colour photo (page 61)

Serve for main meal	Cook at Reg 5
Serve with rice, salad	190°C
Serves 4	Time 50–60 minutes

Ingredients

4 chicken portions
6 tablespoons fresh chopped mint
4 tablespoons ground coriander
2 teaspoons ground cumin
Black pepper
Small pot natural yogurt

Method

1   Prick the chicken all over with a sharp knife.
2   Mix the spices, a pinch of black pepper, the mint and the yogurt together.
3   Pour the spice mixture over the chicken. Leave in the refrigerator overnight or for as long as possible to marinate (allow the flavour to soak into the chicken).
4   Heat the oven.
5   Place the chicken in a casserole dish and cook for 30 minutes. Spoon the sauce over the chicken from time to time.
6   After 30 minutes turn the heat down to Reg 4 or 180°C. Cook until the chicken is tender and there is a brown crust.
7   Serve with rice and a salad.

Chicken curry

See colour photo (page 61)

Serve for main meal
Serve with rice and accompaniments (see below)
Serves 2

Ingredients

2 chicken portions
1 small onion
1 level tablespoon wholemeal flour
$\frac{1}{2}$ teaspoon ground ginger
$\frac{1}{2}$ teaspoon turmeric
$\frac{1}{2}$ teaspoon ground cumin
$\frac{1}{2}$ teaspoon ground coriander
$\frac{1}{2}$ teaspoon garam masala
1 tablespoon chopped fresh coriander or parsley
250 ml water + quarter of a stock cube
1 small eating apple
Squeeze of lemon juice
25 g sultanas
1 dessertspoon chutney
100 g brown rice

This makes a very mild curry. If you like it hot, add 1 cm peeled and chopped root ginger and/or half a very small seeded, chopped chilli.

Method

1   Put a shallow serving dish to warm.
2   Peel and chop the onion and apple.
3   Wash and chop the coriander or parsley.
4   Toss the chicken portions in the flour. A quick way to do this is to put the chicken joints in a paper or polythene bag with the flour and shake. (Old flour bags are useful for this.) Place the chicken joints in a large saucepan.
5   Mix the spices to a paste with a little water. Add the rest of the water and the stock cube. Pour into the saucepan and bring to the boil, stirring.
6   Add the onion and apple, sultanas, chutney and lemon juice.

7   Simmer 45–60 minutes, stirring from time to time until the chicken is tender. Test the chicken with the point of a knife.
8   Put the rice into boiling water and boil for 35–40 minutes until it feels tender when squeezed between finger and thumb. Drain.
9   Arrange the rice round the edge of the serving dish. Pour the curry in the centre.
10   Sprinkle with the chopped parsley or coriander.

This dish could also be pressure cooked — cook for 10 minutes at 15 lb pressure.

To use cooked chicken

It will save time if the chicken can be cooked beforehand, and making curry can be a good way to use left-over chicken (or turkey). Cooked chopped chicken or chicken joints may be used instead of fresh chicken:
Add 1 level tablespoon cornflour to the spices.
Do not coat the chicken with flour.
Cook the sauce for 30 minutes, then add the cooked chicken and cook for 15 minutes more.

Garam masala

Garam masala is a hot spicy mixture. It can be bought but you can make your own by grinding the following spices together in a coffee grinder:

1 tablespoon cardamom seeds
5 cm stick cinnamon
1 teaspoon cumin seeds
1 teaspoon black peppercorns
1 teaspoon whole cloves
Quarter of an average sized nutmeg

This makes about 3 tablespoons.
(*Note*: You will need to clean the coffee grinder thoroughly before and after.)

Accompaniments

It is traditional to serve small dishes of accompaniments with curry, e.g.

Chutney or other pickles
Sliced banana in lemon juice
Cucumber sliced in yogurt
Sliced tomatoes
Coconut
Poppadums (grilled until crisp)
Peanuts
Grated carrot

7 Add the milk gradually to the flour mixture,
   stirring with a wooden spoon.
8 Return to the heat and bring to the boil,
   stirring all the time.
9 Add the mushrooms, rabbit and nutmeg
   and simmer gently for 5 minutes.
10 Just before serving stir in the yogurt.
11 Sprinkle with parsley.

Rabbit in parsnip and mushroom sauce

Serve for main meal
Serve with potatoes, fresh vegetables
Serves 4

Ingredients

500 g rabbit pieces
200 g parsnips
1 heaped tablespoon wholemeal flour
50 g polyunsaturated margarine
250 ml skimmed milk
1 teaspoon French mustard
100 g mushrooms
$\frac{1}{4}$ teaspoon grated nutmeg
1 bayleaf
1 tablespoon natural yogurt
Parsley

Method

1 Peel and grate the parsnips.
2 Pressure cook the rabbit and parsnips with
   the bayleaf in enough water or stock to
   cover for 15 minutes at 15 lb pressure.
3 Wash and slice the mushrooms.
4 Wash, dry and chop the parsley.
5 Melt the margarine in a saucepan. Add the
   flour and cook gently together. Remove
   from the heat.
6 Make the milk up to 500 ml with the stock
   from the pressure cooker.

Bean and chilli liver

See colour photo (page 64)

Serve for main meal
Serve with salad, and rice or crisp French bread
Serves 4

Ingredients

1 onion
350 g lamb's liver
1 tablespoon wholemeal flour
1 teaspoon chilli powder
1 teaspoon dried mixed herbs
400 g canned *or* cooked red kidney beans (see
   page 90)
400 g canned *or* fresh tomatoes
Parsley

Method

1 Wash and skin the liver. Slice into thin strips
   about 5 cm long.
2 Peel and chop the onion. Wash, dry and
   chop the parsley.
3 Peel and chop fresh tomatoes.
4 Toss the liver in the flour and chilli.
5 Put the liver into a saucepan. Add the
   tomatoes, gradually, stirring with a wooden
   spoon.
6 Stir in the onion, herbs and kidney beans.
7 Cook 15–20 minutes stirring now and again.
8 Sprinkle with chopped parsley.

Mexican hotpot

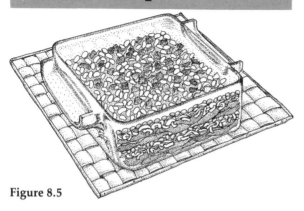

Figure 8.5

Serve for main meal
Serve with jacket
potatoes and a fresh
vegetable
Serves 2

Cook at Reg 4
180°C
Time 30–35 minutes

Ingredients

150 g lamb's liver
1 medium sized onion
1–2 sticks celery
Small can baked beans
50 g bacon
1 tablespoon vegetable oil
Parsley

Method

1 Put the oven on.
2 Wash and dry the liver. Remove the skin
   and any tough parts. Cut into thin strips.
3 Peel and chop the onion.
4 Remove the fat from the bacon and chop or
   snip the bacon into small pieces.
5 Wash and slice the celery thinly.
6 Wash and chop the parsley.
7 Put layers of liver, onion and celery, and
   beans in a casserole dish. Repeat.
8 Sprinkle the chopped bacon over the top.
9 Cover and cook for 30–35 minutes,
   removing the lid for the last 5 minutes to
   crisp the bacon.
10 Sprinkle with the chopped parsley.

Saucy liver and kidneys with herb scones

Serve for main meal
Serve with fresh
vegetable
Serves 4

Cook at Reg 5
190°C
Time 45 minutes

then

Cook at Reg 7
220°C
Time 15–20 minutes

Ingredients

For the casserole

400 g lamb's liver
2 pig's kidneys
25 g wholemeal flour
1 small green pepper
2 carrots
1 onion
Small can tomatoes
250 ml water + half a stock cube

For the herb scones

100 g wholemeal flour
100 g white flour
2 rounded teaspoons baking powder
$\frac{1}{4}$ teaspoon cayenne pepper
$\frac{1}{2}$ teaspoon dried mixed herbs
50 g polyunsaturated margarine
4–6 tablespoons skimmed milk
Parsley

Method

Casserole

1 Put the oven on.
2 Wash and dry the liver. Remove the skin
   and any tough parts. Skin kidneys and
   remove tough parts.
3 Toss the liver and kidneys in the flour.

4   Deseed and chop the pepper. Peel and chop the onion. Peel and slice the carrots.
5   Put the liver in a casserole dish. Gradually add the water and stock cube, stirring with a wooden spoon.
6   Put the pepper, onions and carrots into the casserole dish.
7   Add tomatoes.
8   Cover and cook for 45 minutes.

Scones

9   Put the flour and baking powder into a mixing bowl.
10 Rub fat in with finger tips. Add the herbs and cayenne pepper.
11 Add enough milk to give a soft dough.
12 Shape into a circle the size of the casserole dish (about 15 cm). Cut almost through, into 8 triangles.
13 Turn the oven up. Place the scone mixture onto the top of the casserole and cook for 15–20 minutes until golden brown.
14 Wash, dry and chop the parsley. Sprinkle over the top.

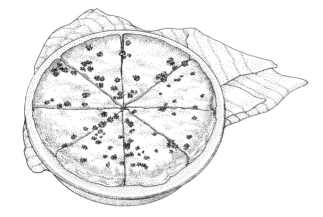

Figure 8.6

Apple topped kidneys

See colour photo (page 64)

Serve for main meal   Cook at Reg 7
Serves 4   220°C
                             Time 20 minutes

                             then

                             Cook at Reg 3
                                  160°C
                             Time 60 minutes

Ingredients

400 g pig's kidneys
1 onion
1 rounded tablespoon wholemeal flour
125 ml cider
$\frac{3}{4}$ teaspoon ground cinnamon
3 tomatoes
25 g currants
200 g brown rice
500 ml water
1 egg
1 eating apple
Black pepper
A little polyunsaturated margarine

Method

1   Put the oven on.
2   Skin the kidneys and cut into thick slices. Toss the kidneys in the flour with a pinch of black pepper.
3   Peel and slice the onion.
4   Peel and slice the tomatoes.
5   Place the kidneys in a saucepan. Gradually add the cider. Bring to the boil stirring all the time.
6   Add the onion, tomatoes, currants and two-thirds of the cinnamon.
7   Pour into a shallow casserole dish. Cover with a lid or foil and cook in the centre of the oven for 20 minutes, then turn down the oven to Reg 3 or 160°C and continue cooking for 1 hour or until the kidneys are cooked.

8   While the kidneys are cooking boil the rice until just tender. Drain and rinse with boiling water.
9   Lightly beat the egg and add to the rice with a pinch of black pepper.
10 Heat the grill. Spoon the rice on top of the kidneys.
11 Core the apple and slice thinly. Arrange slices on top of the rice.
12 Dot with the margarine and sprinkle the cinnamon over.
13 Grill until the apples are browned.

Chilli pasta

See colour photo (page 65)

Serve for main meal
Serve with salad or fresh vegetables
Serves 4

Pressure cook 25 minutes *or* cook on the top of the cooker for 1 hour

Ingredients

400 g stewing steak
2 small onions
Half a green pepper or 1 small one
25 g wholemeal flour
450 ml water + half a stock cube
1 level tablespoon chilli powder
1 level teaspoon oregano and basil, mixed
100 g canned *or* cooked red kidney beans (see page 90)
200 g wholemeal pasta shapes
Parsley

Chilli powder is dried chilli pepper. It gives a dish a hot flavour so cut down the amount if you do not like your food too hot. These peppers are small and pointed in shape and start off green, turning red when ripe. Fresh green chillies are imported from Kenya and are used in many Indian dishes.

Method

1   Put a shallow serving dish to warm.
2   Cut the beef into 2 cm cubes.
3   Peel and chop the onion.
4   Wash, core and remove the pips from the pepper. Chop.
5   Toss the meat in the flour and chilli powder.
6   Put the meat in a saucepan and add the water gradually, stirring with a wooden spoon. Add the stock cube and herbs and bring to the boil, stirring.
7   Add the onion and pepper.
8   Simmer gently for 1 hour. This dish could also be pressure cooked for 25 minutes at 15 lb pressure.
9   Stir in the kidney beans and heat through.
10 Cook the pasta for 10–20 minutes, depending on the shape (see instructions on packet), until rubbery when squeezed between finger and thumb.
11 Wash, dry and chop the parsley.
12 Drain the pasta and spread over serving dish. Pour the meat into the middle.
13 Sprinkle the chopped parsley over the meat.

Spaghetti bolognese

Serve for main meal
Serve with parmesan cheese
Serves 4

Ingredients

400 g minced beef
2 onions
Large can of tomatoes
1 tablespoon wholemeal flour
150 ml water + half a stock cube
1 teaspoon mixed herbs or basil
1 tablespoon tomato purée
2 carrots
200 g wholemeal spaghetti

Method

1 Put a large flat serving dish to warm.
2 Peel and chop the onions and carrots.
3 Put the mince and onions in a large saucepan and cook gently together for 5–6 minutes.
4 Sprinkle the flour in. Add the tomatoes, carrots, tomato purée, stock cube and herbs and 150 ml water.
5 Bring to the boil and simmer gently for 30–45 minutes.
6 Bring a large pan of water to the boil. Hold the spaghetti in the pan and push it down into the water as it softens.
7 Boil for 20 minutes until it feels rubbery when pressed between finger and thumb.
8 Drain the spaghetti and spread over the serving dish.
9 Pour the bolognese sauce into the centre.
10 Serve parmesan cheese separately in a small bowl.

Spaghetti is only one form of **pasta**, which is made from flour, water and sometimes eggs.

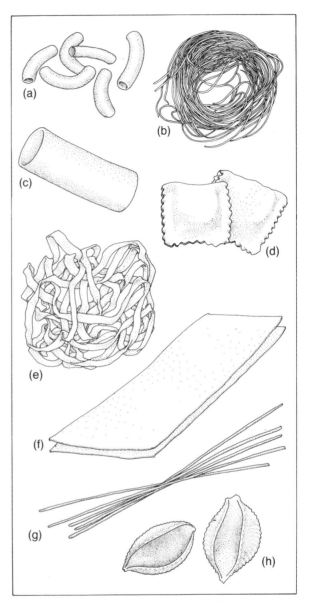

Figure 8.7 How many of these types of pasta can you name? (Answers on page 181)

Beef stew with corn and tomatoes

Serve for main meal
Serve with duchesse or jacket potatoes and fresh vegetables
Serves 4

Pressure cook for 25 minutes

Ingredients

4 tablespoons paprika
400 g stewing steak
1 medium sized onion
200 g can tomatoes
450 ml water + half a stock cube
1 teaspoon dried thyme
1 bay leaf
Shake of black pepper
2 carrots
Large can of sweetcorn
1 level tablespoon cornflour
2–3 sprigs of parsley

Paprika is an orangy-red spice that comes from the dried sweet pepper, grown originally in Hungary. It has a mild flavour.

Method

1 Put a serving casserole dish to warm.
2 Peel and chop the onion. Peel and slice the carrot. Wash, dry and chop the parsley.
3 Cut the beef into 4 cm cubes.
4 Sprinkle the paprika onto a plate. Roll the beef cubes in it until they are well coated.
5 Place the beef, onions, tomatoes, thyme, bayleaf, pepper and carrots, together with any remaining paprika, into the pressure cooker.
6 Add the water and stock cube.
7 Put on the lid and heat until steam escapes. Put the 15 lb weight on and bring up to pressure.
8 Turn the heat down until steam escapes slowly. Pressure cook for 25 minutes.

9 Remove from heat and reduce the pressure.
10 Mix the cornflour with a little cold water Add some of the gravy from the pressure cooker and mix well.
11 Add the sweetcorn and cornflour mixture to the pressure cooker.
12 Return to the heat and bring back to the boil, stirring.
13 Pour into serving dish.
14 Sprinkle the parsley on top.

Mediterranean peppers

See colour photo (page 65)

Serve for main meal	Cook at Reg 5
Serve with rice, salad	190°C
Serves 2	Time 40 minutes

Ingredients

2 large green peppers
1 medium sized onion
150 g minced beef
25 g mushrooms
Small can baked beans *or* kidney beans, *or* use
    200 g cooked kidney beans (see page 90)
1 tablespoon tomato purée
$\frac{1}{2}$ teaspoon basil
Shake of black pepper
100 g brown rice
Parsley

Method

1 Put the oven on. Grease an ovenproof dish. Put a shallow serving dish to warm.
2 Cut off the tops of the peppers and remove the seeds. Trim the bottoms so that they will stand up.
3 Bring a saucepan of water to the boil. Put the peppers in, leave for 3 minutes, then put into cold water.
4 Peel and chop the onion. Wash and slice the mushrooms.
5 Put the mince and onions into a saucepan

and cook gently together for about 10 minutes.

6 Add the mushrooms, beans, tomato purée, basil and pepper, and bring to the boil.

7 Stand the peppers in the dish and fill with the meat mixture. If there is too much to fill the peppers cook the remainder separately in a small ovenproof dish.

8 Cover and cook for 40 minutes.

9 While the peppers are cooking bring a saucepan of water to the boil and put the rice in. Cook 35–40 minutes until tender when squeezed between finger and thumb.

10 Drain the rice and spread on the serving dish. Place the peppers in the middle. Serve any extra meat mixture round the peppers.

11 Garnish with a sprig of parsley.

Italian cobbler

Serve for main meal	Cook at Reg 6
Serve with fresh	200°C
vegetables	Time 15–20 minutes
Serves 4	(+ 25 minutes simmering)

Ingredients

400 g minced beef
1 small onion
1 level tablespoon wholemeal flour
50 g mushrooms
Small can tomatoes
75 ml water
Shake black pepper
Parsley

For the cobbler topping

100g wholemeal flour
100 g white flour
2 teaspoons baking powder
1 level teaspoon oregano *or* a pinch of mixed herbs
50 g polyunsaturated margarine
7 tablespoons skimmed milk + a little extra to glaze

Method

1 Put the oven on.

2 Peel and chop the onion. Wash and slice the mushrooms.

3 Put the mince and onions in a large saucepan and cook gently for 5–6 minutes.

4 Sprinkle in the flour.

5 Add the water, tomatoes, mushrooms and pepper and bring to the boil, stirring.

6 Simmer gently for 25 minutes.

To make cobbler topping (steps 7–10)

7 Rub the margarine into the flour with finger tips.

8 Add herbs.

9 Add enough milk to form a soft dough.

10 Roll out and cut into nine 6 cm circles (see page 133).

11 Pour the meat mixture into an ovenproof casserole dish.

12 Arrange the scones, overlapping, on top around the edge. Brush with milk.

13 Bake half-way down the oven for 15–20 minutes or until golden brown.

14 Garnish with a sprig of parsley.

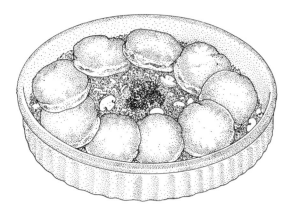

Figure 8.8

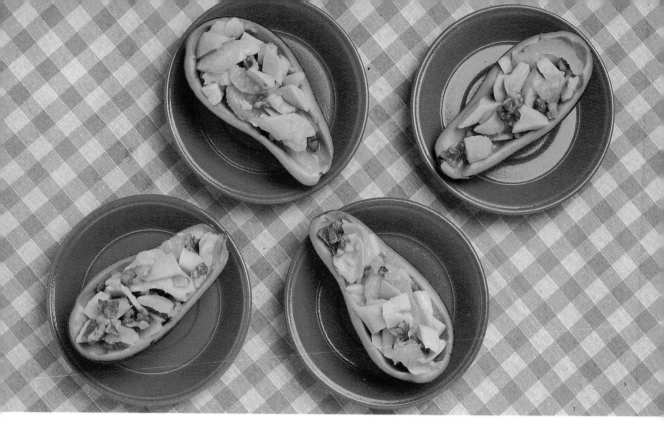

Avocado, orange and nut cocktail (page 44) ▲

Hummus with crudités (page 45) ▼

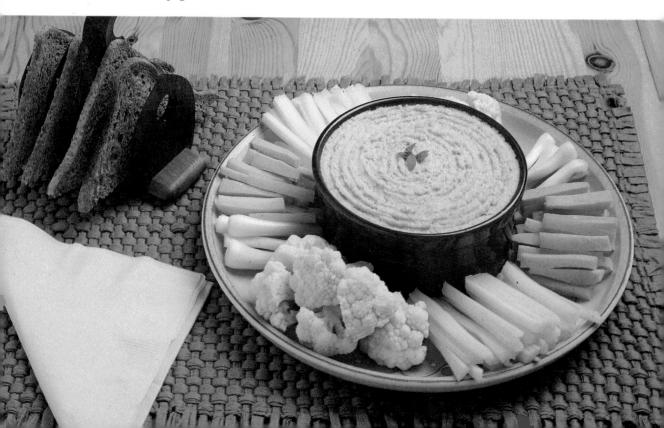

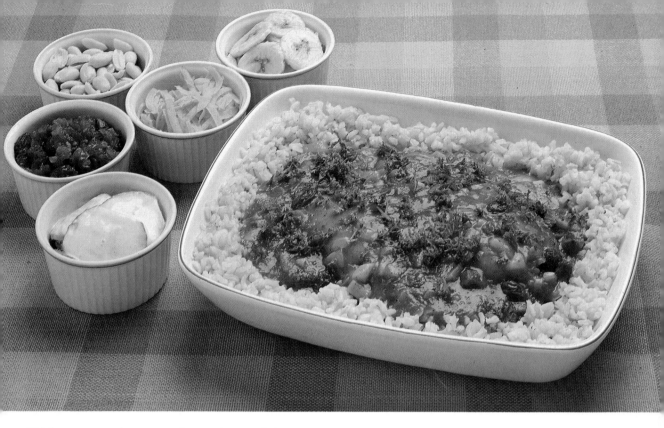

Chicken curry and accompaniments (page 52) ▲

Spicy chicken (page 51) ▼

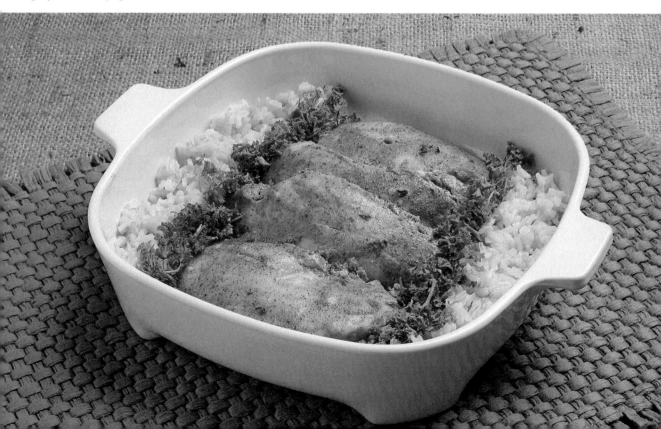

Hereford pie

Serve for main meal
Serve with gravy or
tomato sauce, fresh
vegetables
Serves 4

Cook at Reg 6
　　200°C
Time 30 minutes

then

Cook at Reg 3
　　150°C
Time 10–15 minutes

Ingredients

For the pastry

100 g wholemeal flour
100 g white flour
100 g polyunsaturated margarine
Water to mix

For the filling

200 g minced beef
100 g packet frozen mixed vegetables
2–3 sprigs of parsley
Few drops Worcestershire sauce
1 level tablespoon wholemeal flour

This pie has pastry only on the top, not on the
bottom, to cut down on fat.

Method

1　Put the oven on.
2　Make the shortcrust pastry (see page 128).

To cover the top of a pie dish

3　Roll pastry out to
　the size of the pie
　dish plus the rim
　again.

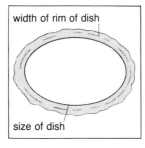
width of rim of dish
size of dish

4　Trim the pastry
　round the dish
　and cut the extra
　into three pieces.

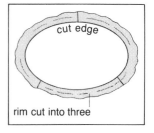
cut edge
rim cut into three

5　Damp the rim of
　the dish and place
　the three pieces
　round the rim
　with the cut side
　outside.

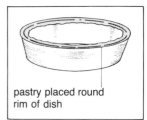
pastry placed round
rim of dish

6　Wash, dry and chop the parsley.

7　Mix all the filling ingredients together.
　Spoon into the pie dish.

8　Damp the pastry edge. Using a rolling pin
　pick the pastry top up and lay over the
　filling.

9　Knock back the
　edges together
　with a knife.

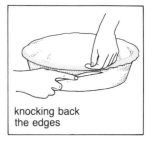
knocking back
the edges

Flute the edges
between finger
and thumb.
Make an air hole
in the top with a
knife.

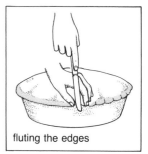
fluting the edges

10　Bake for 30 minutes, then turn the heat
　down for the last 10–15 minutes. The top of
　the pie should be golden and the meat
　cooked.

11　Garnish with parsley.

Moussaka

Serve for main meal
Serve with fresh
vegetables
Serves 4

Cook at Reg 5
190°C
Time 1–1½ hours

Ingredients

300 g minced beef
2 small onions
3–4 sprigs parsley
200 g tomatoes
Shake black pepper
600 g potatoes

For the sauce

12 g polyunsaturated margarine
12 g wholemeal flour
250 ml skimmed milk
1 egg
25 g firm low fat cheese

Method

1 Put the oven on. Grease a casserole dish.
2 Peel and chop the onions and tomatoes. Wash, dry and chop the parsley.
3 Grate the cheese.
4 Put the meat, onions, parsley and tomatoes in a large saucepan and cook gently together for 8 minutes.
5 Scrub and peel the potatoes. Slice thinly. (A food processor is good for this.)
6 Put a layer of potatoes in the bottom of the dish, then a layer of the meat mixture. Continue like this finishing with a layer of potatoes.
7 Melt the margarine in a small saucepan. Mix in the flour.
8 Remove from the heat. Stir in the milk *gradually*. Return to the heat and bring to the boil, stirring all the time.
9 Cool slightly. Stir in the beaten egg and cheese.
10 Pour the sauce over the potatoes in the dish.
11 Cook 1½ hours until golden brown.
12 Garnish with a sprig of parsley.

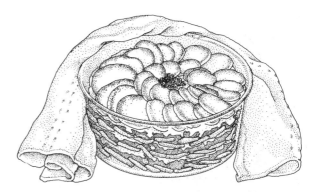

Figure 8.9

Moussaka is a Greek dish and in Greece it would be made with slices of aubergines (which are very cheap there) instead of potatoes, and with lamb rather than beef.

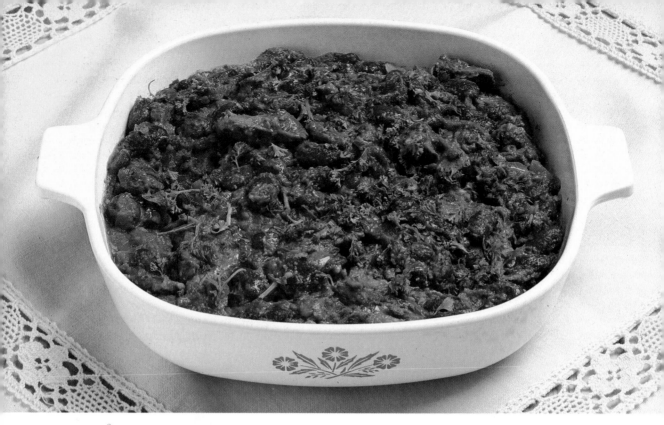

Bean and chilli liver (page 53) ▲

Apple topped kidneys (page 55) ▼

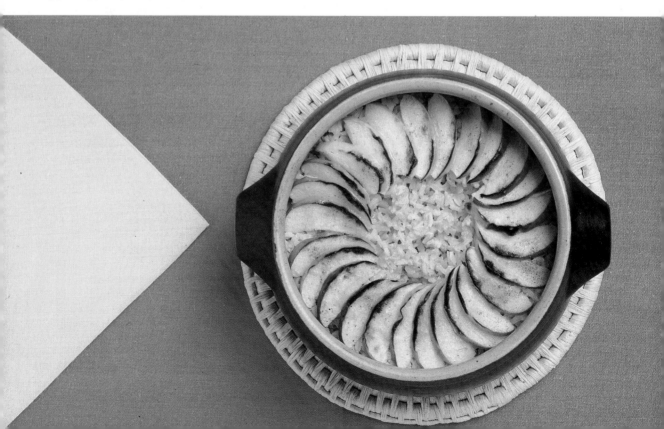

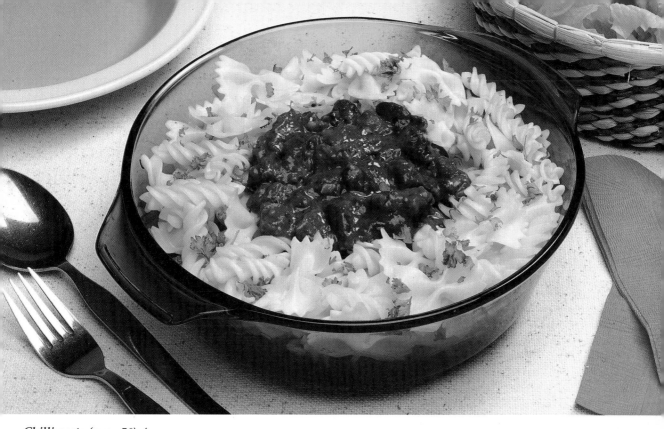

Chilli pasta (page 56) ▲

Mediterranean peppers (page 58) ▼

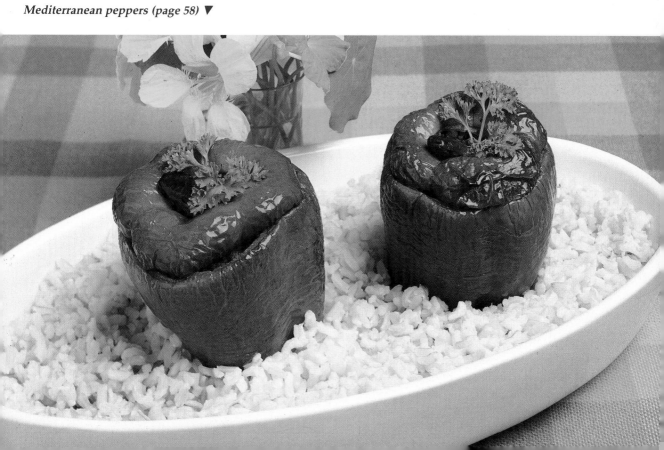

Normandy pork

Serve for main meal
Serve with rice or potatoes and fresh vegetables
Serves 4

Ingredients

4 pork chops
1 medium sized onion
25 g wholemeal flour
450 ml dry cider
2 eating apples
2–3 sprigs parsley
A sprig of thyme or rosemary (or $\frac{1}{2}$ teaspoon
    dried)

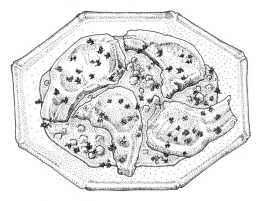

Figure 8.10

Method

1   Put a serving dish to warm.
2   Peel and chop the onion.
3   Wash, dry and chop the parsley and fresh
    herbs.
4   Wipe the chops and cut off fat. Coat with
    flour. An easy way to do this is to put the
    flour and chops in a paper or polythene bag
    (an old flour bag is ideal) and shake
    together.
5   Put the cider in a large shallow frying pan,
    add the onion, chops and herbs.
6   Cover and simmer for 30–40 minutes.

7   Core and dice the apples.
8   Stir into the pan and heat for 3 minutes.
9   Turn into a serving dish.
10 Sprinkle with chopped parsley.

Baked lamb chops with tomatoes and cheese

Serve for main meal   Cook at Reg 3
Serve with potatoes   170°C
and fresh vegetables   Time 1$\frac{1}{2}$ hours
Serves 4

Ingredients

4 loin lamb chops
2 onions
300 g canned tomatoes
Shake of black pepper
$\frac{1}{2}$ teaspoon rosemary
50 g firm low fat cheese
50 g wholemeal bread

Method

1   Put the oven on.
2   Grate the cheese.
3   Make breadcrumbs, using food processor or
    grater.
4   Peel and slice the onions.
5   Place the chops in a single layer in a large
    shallow casserole dish.
6   Put several slices of onion on top of each
    chop.
7   Mix pepper and herbs with tomatoes and
    pour over chops.
8   Mix the cheese and breadcrumbs and scatter
    over the top.
9   Cover and cook until the chops are tender.

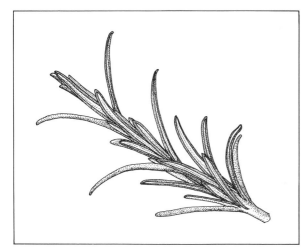

Figure 8.11   Rosemary

Rosemary is a herb which came originally from the Mediterranean. It is an Italian custom to flavour lamb with rosemary.

Braised lamb with apricots

Serve for main meal
Serve with rice or
potatoes and fresh
vegetables
Serves 4

Cook at Reg 5
190°C
Time 1–1½ hours

Ingredients

8 best end *or* middle neck lamb cutlets
2 onions
2 large carrots
2 sticks celery
150 ml water + half a chicken stock cube
50 g tomato purée
10 dried apricots
1 tablespoon wholemeal flour
1 level teaspoon paprika

Method

1   Put the oven on.
2   Wipe and trim fat from meat.
3   Peel and chop onions.
4   Peel and slice carrots.
5   Wash and slice celery thinly.
6   Toss the meat in the flour and paprika.
7   Put the meat in a casserole dish and gradually stir in the water and stock cube, mixing with a wooden spoon.
8   Mix in the tomato purée and apricots, onion, carrots and celery.
9   Cover and cook until the meat is tender. This dish can also be cooked on top of the stove by simmering gently for the same time.
10 Add more liquid if necessary.

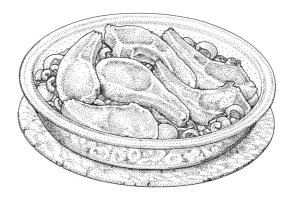

Figure 8.12

Devilled lamb cutlets

Serve for main meal
Serve with rice or potatoes and fresh vegetables
Serves 4

Ingredients

8 best end neck lamb cutlets
2 teaspoons lemon juice
2 level teaspoons dry mustard
1 level teaspoon curry powder
2 level teaspoons fruity sauce

Method

1 Mix lemon juice, mustard, curry powder and
   sauce together.
2 Wipe the cutlets and trim off any fat. Brush
   with half of the sauce.
3 Grill 5–6 minutes.
4 Turn. Brush with the rest of the sauce.
5 Grill 5–6 minutes.

In this recipe the sauce keeps the meat moist so
there is no need to brush with fat.

Hotpot

Serve for main meal   Cook at Reg 6
Serve with fresh   200°C
vegetable   Time 1½ hours
Serves 4

Ingredients

400 g middle neck lamb
400 g potatoes
1 large onion
200 g carrots
500 ml water + half a stock cube
Shake black pepper
2 bayleaves

Method

1 Put the oven on.
2 Peel and chop the onion. Peel and slice the
   carrots.
3 Peel and slice potatoes thinly. N.B. A food
   processor is very useful for preparing the
   vegetables for this dish.
4 Dissolve the stock cube in boiling water.
5 Put the lamb at the bottom of a casserole
   dish.
6 Build up layers of onion, carrot, and
   potatoes alternately, adding the
   bayleaves, and finishing with a layer of
   potatoes.
7 Pour stock over so that it comes three-
   quarters of the way up the dish.
8 Cover with a piece of greased greaseproof
   paper, then a lid, and cook for about an
   hour.
9 Remove the lid, but leave the paper on, for
   the last half hour to crispen the potatoes.

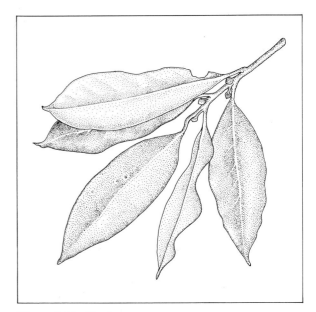

Figure 8.13   Bayleaves

Bayleaves are the tough leaves of the bay tree.
They are dried and added to meat dishes to
provide flavour.

Fish dishes

Fish

Fish is another good source of protein. It is very easy to digest and is therefore suitable for invalids or people with digestive problems.

There are three types of fish:

(a) white fish, which contain less than 5% fat in their flesh, e.g. cod, whiting, plaice, haddock, sole, coley (saithe), halibut;

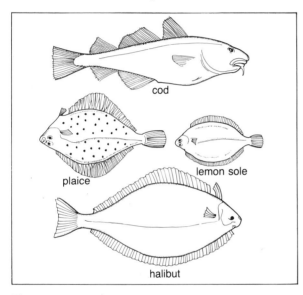

Figure 8.14 White fish

(b) oily fish, which contain more than 5% fat in their flesh, e.g. mackerel, sardine, herring, pilchard, sprat, salmon;

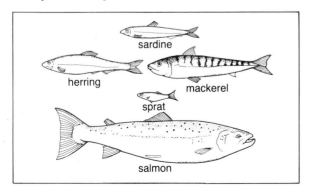

Figure 8.15 Oily fish

(c) shellfish, e.g. lobster, crab, shrimps, cockles, mussels, winkles.

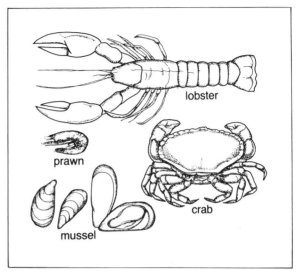

Figure 8.16 Shellfish

Oily fish contain vitamins A and D in their fat. In white fish these vitamins are only in the liver oil, for example in cod liver oil.

The fat in oily fish is polyunsaturated fat (PUFA). We need some PUFA fats to help reduce cholesterol so it is a good idea to include some oily fish regularly in the diet.

Fish contains calcium in the bones but you will only have this if the bones of the fish are eaten, e.g. in canned salmon. Fish also contain iodine and fluoride.

Preserving fish

Fish goes off very quickly. It can be preserved so that it lasts longer, by freezing, canning, smoking, salting or drying.

Smoking is carried out over wood smoke which develops the smokey taste and preserves the fish. Examples of smoked fish are:

Haddock
This is sold as smoked haddock, golden cutlets or finnan haddock. It goes a lovely golden colour.

Mackerel

This is sold as smoked mackerel. It is usually cooked and smoked.

Salmon

This is sold as smoked salmon. It is very expensive.

Herring

These are preserved in several ways:
(a) Kippers — herring are split open, soaked in brine (salt solution) and then smoked;
(b) Buckling — the heads are removed, the fish are salted, smoked and cooked at the same time;
(c) Bloaters — the fish are salted whole, then smoked;
(d) Roll mops — the fish are filleted, soaked in vinegar and brine for 10 days, rolled with pickling spices and pickled.

These are all very salty versions of fish. Dried fish is also very salty.
Smoked fish, like all salty foods, can increase blood pressure, so only eat a little and not too often.

Cooking fish

Fish has less connective tissue than meat and is easier to make tender and quicker to cook. Most methods of cooking can be used. The microwave oven is very useful for cooking fish. It cooks it extremely quickly preserving all the flavour; in fact it is possible to overcook unless you are careful.

Choosing fish

Because it needs to be very fresh, fish should be chosen with care. The fish should have:
(a) bright eyes;
(b) plump firm flesh;
(c) bright firm scales;

(d) moist skin (beware the fishmonger who scatters a lot of water around);
(e) a fresh sea smell;
(f) bright red gills, not sunk in.

Fish can be bought as whole fish, or filleted (boned), or as steaks or cutlets (larger fish cut up).

Filleting fish

A whole fish

1 Scrape off the scales.

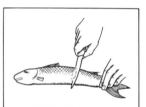

2 Cut off the tail and fins.

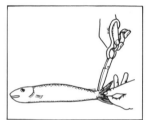

3 Cut off the head just below the gills.

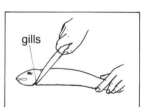

4 Cut open.

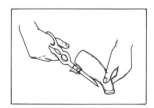

5 Scrape out the inside.

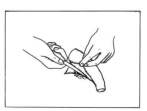

6   Wash.

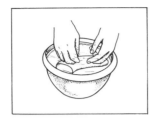

7   Dry on kitchen
paper.

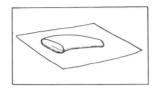

8   Spread the fish
out, skin side up.
Press down along
the backbone with
your thumbs.

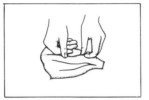

9   Turn over. Loosen
the backbone with
a knife and
remove.

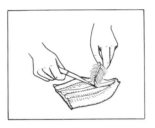

10   Wash and dry.

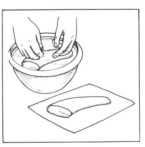

A flat fish

1   Mark round the fillets with a sharp knife.

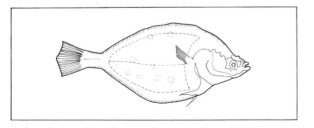

2   Slice the fillet from the bone and remove.

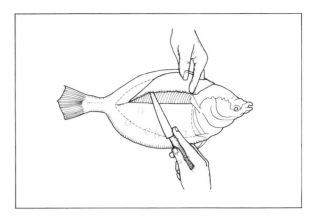

3   Holding the pointed end of the fillet between
your finger and thumb, slide a knife between
the fish and the skin. Remove the skin.

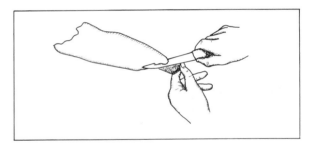

4   Repeat for the second fillet.

5   Wash and dry.

The fish recipes

In any of these recipes the fish can be cooked in
the microwave instead of steaming. Cook,
covered, in a little milk for 8–10 minutes.

Cod or Whiting Eastern style

See colour photo (page 88)

Serve for main meal
Serve with rice or potatoes and fresh vegetables
Serves 4

Ingredients

400 g whiting *or* cod fillet
1 tablespoon lemon juice
1 tablespoon vegetable oil
1 tablespoon wholemeal flour
1 onion
100 g tomatoes
1 level tablespoon mild curry powder
1 level tablespoon apple chutney
4 tablespoons water
Shake of black pepper
Parsley

Method

1 Put a shallow serving dish to warm.
2 Remove the skin from the fish. Cut the fish into large pieces.
3 Sprinkle with lemon juice and leave for 15 minutes.
4 Peel and chop the tomatoes.
5 Peel and chop the onion.
6 Place the flour and pepper on a plate. Coat the fish with flour.
7 Heat the oil in a frying pan. Fry the fish lightly until brown. Remove from the pan.
8 Add onion and curry powder to the pan. Fry gently together for 4 minutes.
9 Add the chutney, water and tomatoes and bring to the boil.
10 Add the fish. Cook until the fish is tender (about 10 minutes).
11 Wash dry and chop the parsley.
12 Spoon the fish onto serving dish. Sprinkle with parsley.

Fish mornay

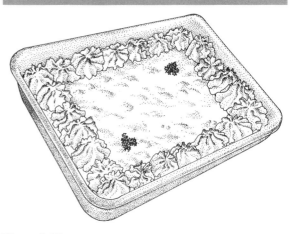

Figure 8.17

Serve for main meal, for invalids
Serve with fresh vegetables
Serves 2

Ingredients

100 g cod *or* coley
250 ml skimmed milk
25 g polyunsaturated margarine
25 g wholemeal flour
50–75 g firm low fat cheese
200 g potatoes + a little extra skimmed milk
2 sprigs parsley

Method

1 Put a casserole dish to warm.
2 Peel potatoes. Cut into small pieces. Place in a pan of boiling water. Place a covered plate on top with the fish on to steam (see Figure 8.22) for about 20 minutes until the fish and potatoes are tender.
3 Grate the cheese.
4 Wash and dry the parsley.
5 Make a roux sauce (see page 114) with the margarine, milk and flour.
6 Stir in the grated cheese, saving a little for the top.
7 Mash the potatoes with milk until smooth. Pipe round the edge of the dish.
8 Place the cooked fish in the dish.

9 Pour the sauce over.
10 Sprinkle the remaining cheese on top. Grill until golden brown.
11 Garnish with sprigs of parsley.

Fish pie

Serve for main meal
Serve with fresh vegetables
Serves 4

Ingredients

300 g haddock *or* cod *or* coley
25 g polyunsaturated margarine
25 g wholemeal flour
250 ml skimmed milk
50 g firm low fat cheese
Shake of black pepper
3–4 sprigs of parsley
1 egg
2 tomatoes

For the topping

600 g potatoes
4 tablespoons skimmed milk

Method

1 Peel the potatoes, cut into small pieces. Place in a pan of boiling water. Place a covered plate on top with the fish on to steam (see Figure 8.19) for about 15 minutes or until the fish is tender. The potatoes may need to be left on for another 5–10 minutes.
2 Grate the cheese. Peel and slice the tomato.
3 Wash, dry and chop the parsley, saving one piece whole for a garnish.
4 Hard boil the egg, plunge into cold water. Shell and slice.
5 Make a roux sauce (see page 114) with the margarine, flour and milk.

6 Drain the fish, remove skin and flake with a fork.
7 Add the cheese, pepper, fish, tomato and egg to the sauce and stir gently.
8 Mash the potatoes with milk until smooth. Pipe over the fish. Brown under the grill.
9 Garnish with parsley.

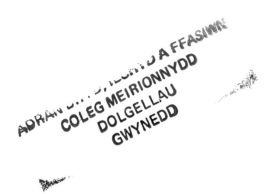

Figure 8.18

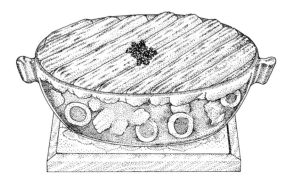

Fish and cheese crumble

Serve for main meal
Serve with potatoes,
fresh vegetables
Serves 4

Cook at Reg 4
180°C
Time 20 minutes

Ingredients

300 g cod *or* coley *or* haddock fillet
250 ml skimmed milk
25 g polyunsaturated margarine
25 g wholemeal flour
75 g firm low fat cheese
2 eggs
Shake of black pepper
2 sprigs parsley

For the topping

100 g wholemeal flour
50 g polyunsaturated margarine

Method

1 Put the oven on.
2 Hard boil the eggs. Cook the fish on a covered plate on top of the egg pan (see Figure 8.19) until tender.
3 Grate the cheese. Wash and dry the parsley.
4 Drain the fish. Make the liquid left up to 250 ml with milk. Remove any skin from the fish and flake.
5 Place the fish in a shallow casserole dish. Arrange sliced hard boiled eggs on top.
6 Make a roux sauce with the margarine, flour and milk (see page 114).
7 Add half the cheese, and pepper to the sauce. Pour over the fish.
8 Rub the fat into the flour for the topping. Mix in the rest of the cheese.
9 Sprinkle over the fish.
10 Bake for 20 minutes. The top may be browned under the grill if liked.
11 Garnish with parsley.

Kedgeree

See colour photo (page 88)

Serve for main meal
Serve with fresh
vegetables
Serves 4

Cook at Reg 3
170°C
Time 30 minutes

Ingredients

150 g brown rice
250 g smoked haddock
2 eggs
25 g polyunsaturated margarine
8 tablespoons skimmed milk
Parsley, tomato to garnish

Method

1 Put the oven on. Grease a casserole dish.
2 Put the eggs to hard boil for 10 minutes.
3 Half fill a saucepan with hot water. Add the rice. Cook for 40 minutes or until tender. Place the fish with a little water or milk on a plate with the saucepan lid on top, on top of the saucepan. Steam for about 10 minutes until tender.

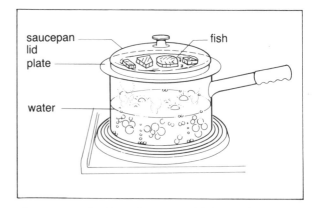

Figure 8.19 Cooking the rice and fish together saves fuel.

4 Rinse the rice with boiling water, in a sieve.
5 Drain the fish, remove skin and bones. Flake with a fork.
6 Plunge the eggs into cold water, shell and chop roughly.
7 Melt the margarine in a saucepan. Add the rice, fish and egg. Mix in the milk.
8 Put in the casserole and cook in the oven for 30 minutes.
9 Skin and slice the tomato. Wash and chop the parsley. Place the tomato on the dish 10 minutes before it comes out of the oven. Sprinkle with parsley before serving.

Kedgeree was originally served as a breakfast dish, but is now served more often for a main meal.

Pour over the cider, bayleaf and spices.
6 Cook until tender. Allow to cool in the liquid.

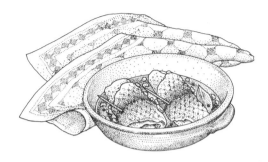

Figure 8.20

Cider soused herrings

Serve for main meal   Cook at Reg 3
Serve with salad   170°C
Serves 2   Time 1 hour

Ingredients

2 herrings
1 small onion
200 ml cider
1 bayleaf
Black pepper
1 teaspoon mixed pickling spice (*or* 6 peppercorns and 2 cloves)
Cocktail sticks

Method

1 Put the oven on.
2 Peel and chop the onion.
3 Remove the heads and fillet the herrings (see page 70).
4 Sprinkle with pepper. Roll up the skin side outside, beginning at the head end. Fasten with cocktail sticks.
5 Place in an ovenproof dish. Add the onion.

Baked stuffed herrings

Serve for main meal   Cook at Reg 5
Serve with sauce   190°C
(e.g. parsley, tomato,   Time 30–40 minutes
mustard), potatoes,
fresh vegetable
Serves 2

Ingredients

2 herrings
For the stuffing

50 g wholemeal bread
Half a beaten egg
3–4 sprigs parsley
$\frac{1}{2}$ teaspoon mixed chopped herbs
Grated rind of half a lemon
Shake of black pepper

Method

1 Put the oven on.
2 Clean and fillet the fish (see page 70). The head may be removed or left on.
3 Make breadcrumbs by grating or using the food processor. Wash, dry and chop the parsley.

4   Mix all the stuffing ingredients together in a small basin.

5   Spread each herring with stuffing. Fold in half.

6   Lay in an ovenproof dish.

7   Cover with greased paper and cook until tender.

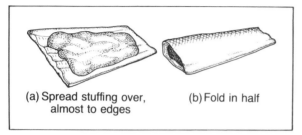

(a) Spread stuffing over, almost to edges

(b) Fold in half

Figure 8.21   Stuffing the herring

Cheese dishes

What is cheese?

Cheese is one of the earliest foods we know of. It is thought that Arabian nomads first made cheese by accident when they carried milk in bags made from the stomachs of animals. The bags were not cleaned very well and the rennin (an enzyme found in the stomach) would have curdled the milk.

Cheese is made, today, by souring milk with an acid 'starter' and then adding rennet. This causes the milk to split into curds and whey. The curd, or solid part, is used to make cheese. Salt is added and the curd is pressed into moulds and left to mature or ripen. If a very hard cheese is wanted the curd is pressed to squeeze out all the moisture, but for a soft cheese some of the whey is left in the cheese.

Because cheese is made from milk it has more or less the same nutrients. It is a good source of protein, calcium and vitamin A, but it also has a lot of fat. Cheese is:

> one-third protein
> one-third fat
> one-third water

and it is very salty. Cream cheese contains the most fat as it is made from cream rather than milk. Processed cheese is made from melting and mixing other cheeses with colouring and flavouring added. Cottage cheese contains the least fat. It is made from skimmed milk. Edam is another lower fat cheese and there are many 'low fat' cheeses being developed now to help us cut down on eating fat.

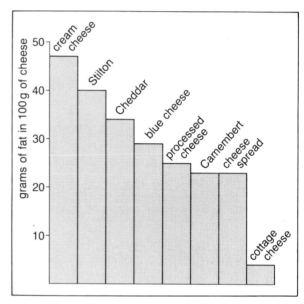

Figure 8.22   The amount of fat in different kinds of cheese. Cottage cheese has by far the least fat (only 4 g in 100 g cheese). Do not forget that although processed cheese and cheese spread look lower in fat than cheddar or blue cheese, they may also contain additives and colouring, and it is best to avoid too many of these.

British cheeses

Hard cheeses: Cheddar, Derby, Cheshire, Double Gloucester, Leicester

Lightly pressed cheeses: Caerphilly, Lancashire, Wensleydale

Blue veined cheeses: (produced by injecting the cheese with harmless bacteria which grow in the air spaces) Stilton, Lymeswold, Melbury

Acid curd cheeses: curd cheese, cottage cheese

Processed cheeses

Cream cheeses

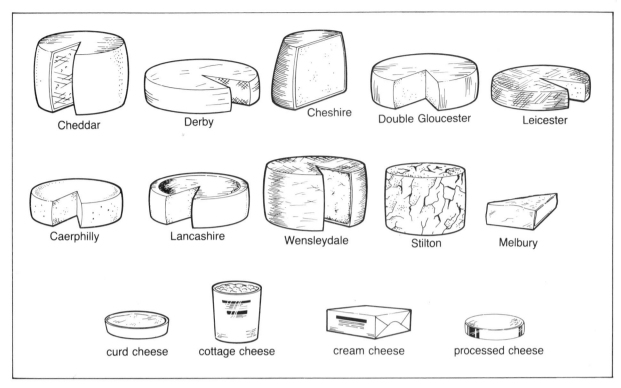

Figure 8.23   British cheeses

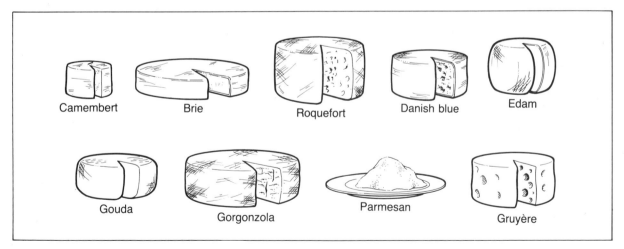

Figure 8.24   Foreign cheeses

Foreign cheeses

France: Camembert, Brie, Roquefort
Denmark: Danish Blue
Holland: Edam, Gouda
Italy: Gorgonzola, Parmesan
Switzerland: Gruyère

Cooking with cheese

Cheese can be used in cooking:
(a) in main dishes, e.g. savoury flans;
(b) in snacks, e.g. Welsh rarebit, Cheese omelette;
(c) to flavour sauces;
(d) grated on salads, in sandwich fillings;
(e) as a garnish for soups, meat sauces, cauliflower cheese, etc.;
(f) as a dessert in cheesecakes;
(g) in shortcrust pastry, scones.
Cheese can be rather indigestible, especially when cooked. This is because each bit of protein is coated with fat which forms a waterproof covering and stops digestion taking place in the stomach.

To make cheese more digestible

1 Grate or shred to break the cheese down.
2 Add strongly flavoured ingredients like mustard or vinegar. This gets the digestive juices going.
3 Avoid overcooking or the protein in the cheese will harden.
4 Serve the cheese with a starchy food — bread, pastry, potatoes. The starch will absorb some of the fat.
5 Do not eat cheese late at night if you find it difficult to digest.

Storage

1 Store cheese in a cold place.
2 Wrap in foil or polythene to prevent drying out.

3 In the refrigerator keep in a covered plastic box to avoid drying out.
4 Curd, cottage and cream cheese will not keep more than a few days. Hard cheeses keep longest.
5 Cheese can be frozen, but it tends to be crumbly when it is taken out of the freezer.

Cheese recipes

See also Cheese omelette
            Savoury supper dish
            Surprise potatoes
            Crisp tuna casserole
            Fish mornay
            Fish pie
            Fish and cheese crumble

Savoury flan

Serve for main meal   Cook at Reg 6
Serve with fresh   200°C
vegetables   Time 30 minutes
Serves 4

Ingredients

For the pastry

75 g wholemeal flour
75 g white flour
75 g polyunsaturated margarine
Water to mix

For the sauce

250 ml skimmed milk
25 g wholemeal flour
25 g polyunsaturated margarine
Filling (see opposite)

Fillings

Choose from:

Chicken and mushroom

150 g cooked chicken
100 g mushrooms, washed and sliced
1 medium onion, peeled and chopped
50 g firm low fat cheese, grated

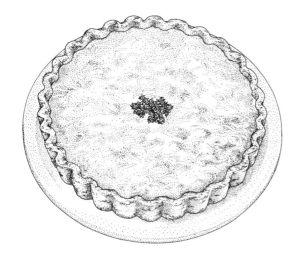

Figure 8.25 Chicken and mushroom flan

Cheese and ham

100 g chopped cooked ham with fat cut off
100 g firm low fat cheese, grated
1 teaspoon mustard
1 teaspoon Worcestershire sauce

Sweetcorn and bacon

75 g firm low fat cheese, grated
Small can sweetcorn
1 teaspoon mustard
100 g bacon with fat cut off, grilled

Salmon

75 g firm low fat cheese, grated
Small tin salmon with juice drained off and skin
    removed, broken up with a fork

Vegetable

Small packet frozen mixed vegetables, cooked
75 g firm low fat cheese, grated

Prawn

Small can prawns (drained) *or* 100 g fresh
    prawns
50 g firm low fat cheese, grated
Hard boiled egg, sliced

Method

1 Put the oven on.
2 Make shortcrust pastry. Line flan ring and
   bake blind (see below).
3 Prepare chosen filling ingredients.
4 Make a roux sauce (see page 114).
5 Stir in the filling ingredients, saving a little of
   the cheese for the top. Pour into the flan
   case.
6 Sprinkle with cheese and brown under the
   grill.
7 The flan may be garnished with parsley or
   peeled, sliced tomato if liked.

To line a flan ring

1 Roll out pastry to
   size of flan ring +
   depth.

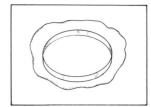

2 Place flan ring on
   baking tray. Lift
   pastry on rolling
   pin and place over
   ring.

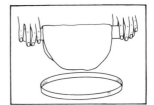

3 Lift edges of pastry
   and press the
   bottom flat. Press
   pastry well into
   corners with
   thumb.

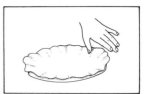

4 Work the extra pastry down the sides of the tin.

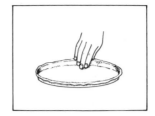

5 Roll off excess.

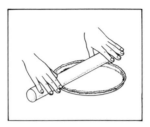

To bake blind:
1 Place a sheet of crumpled greaseproof paper in the flan case and fill with baking beans (pasta or pulses can be used).

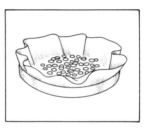

2 Bake at Reg 6 or 200°C for 15 minutes. Remove beans and paper. Return to oven to dry off for 5–10 minutes.

Pizza (scone based)

Serve for main meal, snack, packed meal, buffet
Serve with salad
Serves 4

Cook at Reg 7 220°C
Time 25–30 minutes for one large pizza
15–20 minutes for small individual pizzas

Ingredients

75 g wholemeal flour
75 g white flour
2 teaspoons baking powder
50 g polyunsaturated margarine
150 ml skimmed milk
50 g firm low fat cheese
Topping (see below)

Toppings

Choose from:

Tomato

Small can tomatoes with the juice drained off *or* 200 g peeled, chopped tomatoes
1 onion, peeled and chopped
1 dessertspoon basil or marjoram
(Cook these ingredients together until the onion is soft)

Sardine and tomato

See colour photo (page 89)

Small can tomatoes with the juice drained off *or* 200 g peeled, sliced tomatoes
Can sardines in tomato sauce

Vegetable

50 g mushrooms, washed and chopped
200 g tomatoes, peeled and sliced
75 g sweetcorn, drained

Ham and sweetcorn

75 g ham, chopped
Small can sweetcorn, drained
250 ml skimmed milk, 25 g wholemeal flour, 25 g margarine (made into a roux sauce)
25 g cheese, grated and stirred into the sauce

Fish

150 g kipper fillets *or* smoked haddock,
   cooked on a plate over a saucepan of water
   for 15 minutes
250 ml skimmed milk, 25 g wholemeal flour, 25 g
   margarine (made into a roux sauce)
25 g cheese, grated and stirred into the sauce

Method

1 Put the oven on. Grease a baking tray, and
   for a large pizza a 20 cm flan ring.
2 Prepare the chosen topping.
3 Grate the cheese.
4 Put the flour into a mixing bowl. Rub in the
   fat until the mixture is like fine breadcrumbs.
5 Add enough milk to make a soft (scone)
   dough.
6 For one large pizza roll out to fit the flan ring.
   For small pizzas divide the dough into four
   and roll each piece to a 10 cm circle.
7 Place the pizza on the baking tray and place
   the flan ring over. Press the edge of the
   dough upwards to form a lip to keep the
   topping on the dough.
8 Put on the topping ingredients, finishing
   with the sauce, if you are using one, then the
   cheese.
9 Bake until the top is golden and the scone
   base cooked.

Pizza (pronounced peetza) is an Italian dish, but
there the base is made from bread dough tossed
in the air until thin. There is a recipe for a bread
based pizza on page 148.

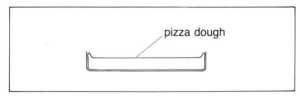

Figure 8.26   The pizza dough is raised at the edges to
stop the topping running off.

Quiche Lorraine

Serve for main meal, buffet, packed meal	Cook at Reg 6 200°C
Serve with salad	Time 10 minutes
Serves 4	then
	Cook at Reg 5 190°C 25–30 minutes

Ingredients

75 g wholemeal flour   150 ml skimmed milk
75 g white flour   2 eggs
1 small onion   50 g firm low fat cheese
2 rashers bacon   Parsley
75 g polyunsaturated
margarine

Method

1 Put the oven on. Grease a baking tray and a
   20 cm flan ring.
2 Rub the fat into the flour until it is like
   breadcrumbs.
3 Add enough cold water to give a stiff
   dough.
4 Roll out to the size of the flan ring + the
   depth. Line the flan ring (see page 79).
5 Trim the fat from the bacon and grill.
6 Peel and chop the onion. Grate the cheese.
   Prepare any of the other fillings to be used.
7 Beat the eggs lightly.
8 Mix in the milk and cheese, saving a little of
   the cheese for the top.
9 Place the bacon (or other filling) and onion
   in the flan case. Spread out.
10 Pour the egg mixture over. Sprinkle cheese
   on top.
11 Bake for 10 minutes, then turn the oven
   down to Reg 5 or 190°C.
12 Bake until golden brown and set. Test by
   inserting a knife into the filling. It should
   part and look set, and the top should feel
   firm.
13 Garnish with a sprig of parsley.

Individual quiches can be made by cooking in small tins for 20–25 minutes. This recipe makes 4.

Quiche Lorraine is a dish from the Lorraine area of France. You can change the filling if you wish. Leaving out the bacon will cut down the fat content, and you could use cottage cheese instead of firm cheese.

Try these for a change:

Cheese and onion quiche

Leave out the bacon.

Cheese and tomato quiche

Add 2–3 tomatoes, peeled and thinly sliced, instead of the bacon.

Cheese and mushroom quiche

Add 100 g mushrooms instead of the bacon. Save some of the mushrooms, sliced, to arrange round the top.

Green and red pepper quiche

Add 1 small green and 1 small red pepper, deseeded and sliced thinly, instead of the bacon.

Egg dishes

Eggs

Eggs are another good source of protein. They are very digestible, especially when lightly cooked, and are often served to people who are getting over an illness.

The white (which forms just over half of the egg) also contains water, B vitamins and a very small amount of fat. The yolk (about 30% of the egg) contains more fat and cholesterol, so it is probably not a good idea to eat too many eggs

each week. The yolk also contains water, and vitamins A, B1, B2, D, E and K. There is also iron in the egg yolk, but the body may not be able to make use of this, so it is no good relying on eggs for iron.

The shell (about 11% of the egg) contains calcium, but as it is not eaten this does not do us any good. The colour of egg shells depends on the food being fed to the chickens and does not make any difference to the nutritional value of the egg inside.

Producing eggs

Hens' eggs are most often used for eating, though duck and goose eggs can be eaten as long as they are very fresh.

Most eggs sold in supermarkets and shops come from battery or deep-litter farms.

Battery farming

Hundreds of hens are kept in cages in large hen houses which are lit and heated. As the eggs are laid they fall onto a conveyor belt and are carried away for checking and grading.

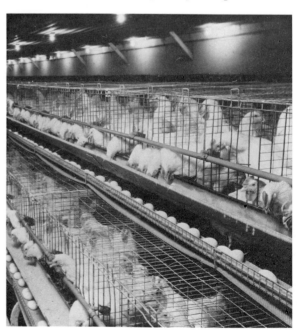

Figure 8.27   Battery hen farming

Deep-litter farming

These hens are kept in large heated sheds, but not in cages. The hens lay in nest boxes.

Some people are uncomfortable about the conditions in which the hens are kept in battery and deep-litter farms and prefer free-range eggs.

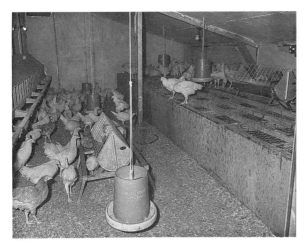

Figure 8.28 Deep-litter hen farming

Free-range farming

Hens are allowed to roam loose and lay their eggs in a hen house. All eggs were once obtained in this way, but it is more economic to produce eggs by battery or deep-litter farming. Free-range eggs can be bought from farms, health food shops and some other shops. They are often more expensive.

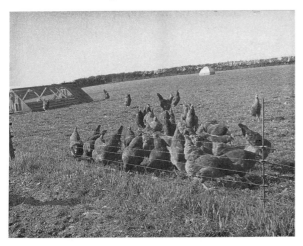

Figure 8.29 Free-range hen farming

Grading eggs

Eggs have had to be graded since 1973 to meet EEC (European Economic Community) regulations.

Size	Weight
1	70 g or more
2	65–70 g
3	60–65 g
4	55–60 g
5	50–55 g
6	45–50 g
7	45 g or less

Eggs are also graded according to quality:

1 Extra High quality eggs — packed within the last seven days.
2 Class A Good quality — these are the eggs we usually buy.
3 Class B Lower quality — may have dirty shells.
4 Class C — usually sold to cake manufacturers as they have weak or damaged shells.

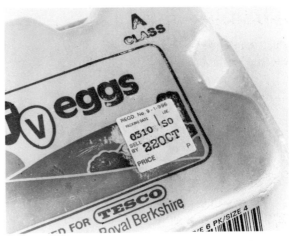

Figure 8.30 Egg cartons should show clearly the egg size and grade and also the country, region, packing station number and date.

Structure of an egg

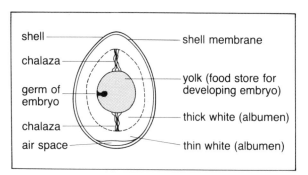

Figure 8.31   Inside an egg

To test for freshness of eggs

1   A fresh egg will have a thick white with only a little thin white around it

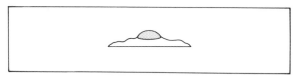

Figure 8.32   Fresh egg

As the egg gets older there will be more thin white.

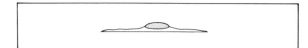

Figure 8.33   Stale egg

2   There will be a bad smell if eggs are very old.
3   You can test whether eggs are fresh by dissolving 50 g salt in 500 ml water and gently putting the unbroken eggs in.

If the eggs are fresh they will stay on their sides at the bottom. If they are less fresh they will stand on end. If they are stale they will float.

This is because the air space in the egg gets larger as the egg gets older — water has evaporated from the white, allowing more air to enter.

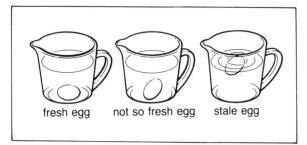

Figure 8.34   Testing eggs for freshness

Uses of eggs

Eggs can be used for a variety of purposes in cooking:
(a)   as a main dish — baked, poached, scrambled, boiled, omelettes etc;
(b)   for thickening custards, sauces, soups, lemon curd;
(c)   for binding together stuffings, rissoles, icing;
(d)   to moisten cakes and help them to keep for longer;
(e)   to hold air in meringues, whisked sponges, soufflés (i.e. a raising agent);
(f)   to glaze pastry, scones;
(g)   as a garnish;
(h)   as a coating, e.g. fish;
(i)   to add extra protein (enrich) but remember you are adding extra cholesterol too!;
(j)   for emulsifying, e.g. in mayonnaise the egg prevents the oil and vinegar from separating.

Storing eggs

1   The shell of an egg is porous (pores are tiny holes), so eggs should be stored away from strong smelling foods like onions.
2   Eggs should be stored with the blunt end on top so that the yolk stays in the middle and the chalaza (see Figure 8.31) does not break.
3   Eggs can be kept in the refrigerator or a cold place. They should be removed from the refrigerator an hour or two before using as they do not whisk well when cold.

4 Eggs may be frozen, but not with the yolk and white together. Separate and freeze separately.

Separating eggs

Many recipes ask for the yolk and white of the egg to be separated. To avoid breaking the yolk use this simple method.

Break the egg onto a plate. Put an egg cup or pastry cutter over the yolk. Pour the white off into a basin.

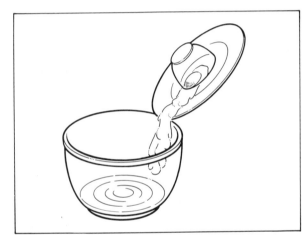

Figure 8.35   Separating an egg

Egg recipes

See also Scrambled eggs
       Poached eggs
       Buck rarebit
       Omelettes
       Devilled eggs
       Quiche Lorraine
       Egg curry

Egg mornay

Serve for main meal, for invalids
Serve with fresh vegetables
Serves 2

Ingredients

2 eggs
250 ml skimmed milk
25 g polyunsaturated margarine
25 g wholemeal flour
50–75 g firm low fat cheese
200 g potatoes + a little extra skimmed milk
2 sprigs parsley

Method

1 Put a casserole dish to warm.
2 Peel potatoes. Cut into small pieces. Place in a pan of boiling water and cook for about 20 minutes until tender.
3 Hard boil the eggs for 10 minutes, then plunge into cold water.
4 Grate the cheese.
5 Wash and dry the parsley.
6 Make a roux sauce (see page 114) with the margarine, flour and milk.
7 Stir in the grated cheese, saving a little for the top.
8 Peel the eggs. Cut in half, lengthwise.
9 Mash the potatoes with milk until smooth.
10 Pipe the potatoes round the edge of the dish.
11 Place the eggs, rounded side up in the dish. Pour the sauce over.
12 Sprinkle the remaining cheese on top. Grill until golden brown.
13 Garnish with the sprigs of parsley.

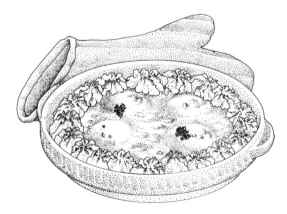

Figure 8.36

Batters

Eggs are one of the ingredients of batters, which are made of milk, flour and eggs.

Basic recipe ingredients

50 g wholemeal flour
50 g white flour
250 ml skimmed milk
1 egg

This will give a pouring batter which could be used for pancakes, Yorkshire pudding or toad in the hole. For a coating batter use only 150 ml milk and use for coating foods such as fish or chicken.

Because most batter dishes are fried or cooked in hot fat it is wise not to eat them too often. Sweet batter dishes are also often covered in lots of sugar. Using wholemeal flour adds some fibre and there is calcium from the milk and protein from the milk and egg. A recipe is given here for one savoury batter dish.

Stuffed pancakes

See colour photo (page 89)

Makes 8–10 pancakes

Ingredients

For the batter

50 g wholemeal flour
50 g white flour
1 egg
250 ml skimmed milk
Pinch black pepper
A little vegetable oil for frying

For the filling

50 g polyunsaturated margarine
50 g wholemeal flour
250 ml skimmed milk
200 g cooked chicken
50 g mushrooms

Parsley

Cooked vegetables may be used in place of cooked chicken if preferred.

Method

To make the batter (steps 1–5)

1   Put a plate to warm in the oven. Put the flour and pepper in a mixing bowl. Make a well in the centre.
2   Break the egg into the flour.
3   Mixing in the middle of the bowl, add the milk gradually and mix in the flour a little at a time, until half the milk is added.
4   Beat until smooth.
5   Stir in the rest of the milk.
6   Brush the bottom of an omelette pan with oil and heat.
7   Give the batter a final stir. Tilting the pan pour in enough batter to just cover the base of the pan. Keep the pancake thin.
8   When golden on the bottom toss to turn, or slip a palette knife under and turn.
9   Cook the other side.
10   When pancakes are cooked slip onto the plate and pile up in the oven, separated by greaseproof paper.
11   Cut the chicken into small pieces. Wash and dry the parsley.
12   Wash and chop the mushrooms.
13   Make the roux sauce (see page 114).
14   Add the chicken and mushrooms and cook gently for 5 minutes.
15   Take each pancake in turn. Put a spoonful of the sauce in the centre and roll up.
16   Place on a serving dish and garnish with parsley.

The pancakes can be made in advance and frozen. They can be taken out of the freezer and filled when needed.

Main meal dishes without meat

Vegetarians

Some people prefer not to eat meat, either all or part of the time. Vegetable dishes can provide variety in the diet and cut down on the cost of expensive meats.

People who never eat meat are called **vegetarians**. People may be vegetarian:

(a) for religious reasons, e.g. Hindus do not eat beef, Jewish people do not eat pork;
(b) to avoid cruelty to animals;
(c) because it is more expensive to rear animals than to use land for crops;
(d) because they do not like the taste of meat;
(e) because they believe that a vegetarian diet is more healthy.

There are two types of vegetarian, lacto vegetarians and vegans.

Foods for lacto vegetarians

Lacto vegetarians will not eat meat, fish or lard. To produce these, animals have to be killed. They *will* eat eggs, milk, cheese, butter, cream and yogurt, which are produced without having to kill animals.

It is possible for lacto vegetarians to buy cheese which has not been made with rennet (which comes from the stomach of the calf). Vegetarian rennet comes from figs. This sort of cheese is usually found in a health food shop.

Lacto vegetarians can get the protein they need from eggs and cheese and also from pulse vegetables (peas, beans, lentils) and nuts, and from soya and its products. Soya beans are particularly high in protein.

Soya products

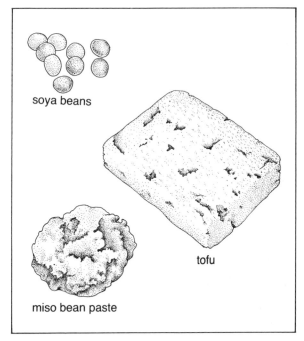

Figure 8.37   Soya products

Soya beans

Miso bean paste

This is fermented soya bean paste. Cooked soya beans and rice have an organism called *Aspergillus oryzae* added. Salt is also added and the mixture is fermented until a paste is formed.

Miso varies in colour from black to white. The darker the colour the more soya beans have been added and less rice. Miso can be made into soups, gravies or added to casseroles.

Savoury miso beans

These are beans rolled from fermented soya beans, ginger and salt. They are eaten as a starter.

Tempeh

This is a cheese made from fermented soya beans. It has a strong smell and taste, a bit like gorgonzola.

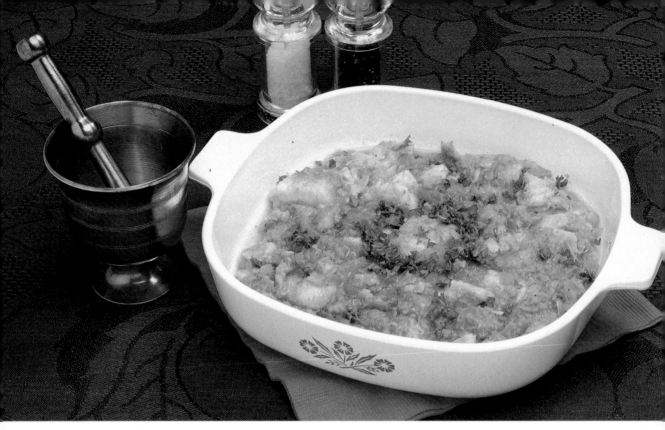

Cod Eastern style (page 72) ▲

Kedgeree (page 74) ▼

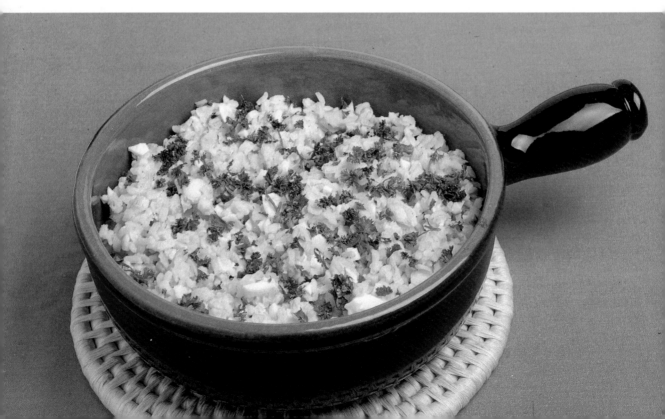

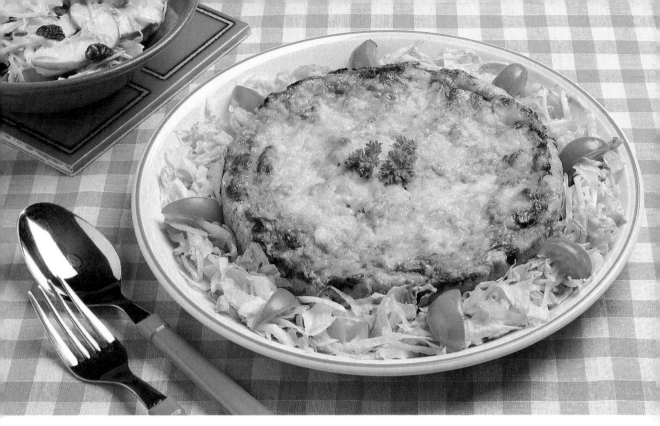

Sardine and tomato pizza (page 80) ▲

Stuffed pancakes (page 86) ▼

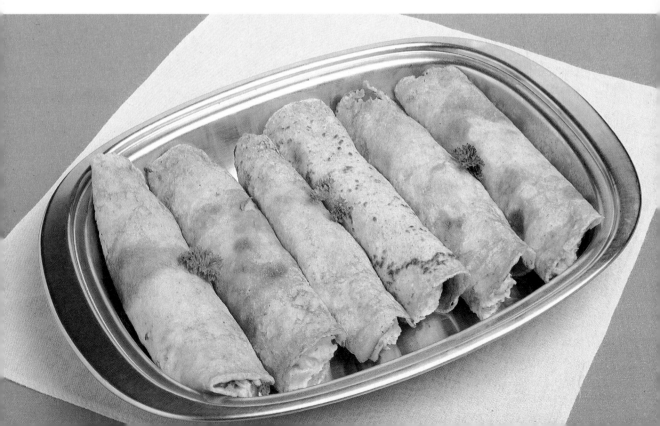

Tofu

This is soya bean curd made by grinding beans and curdling them with powdered gypsum. This has an effect like rennin which is used to make milk into junket.

Tofu has a soft texture and pale cream colour. It is low in fat and calories, but high in protein and can be used in sweet or savoury dishes. Most of the other nutrients needed can also be provided by the foods lacto vegetarians can eat. Sometimes they do not get enough iron as most of our iron comes from meat. There is some in eggs, but the body is not able to use this as easily. If necessary iron tablets could be taken. Most vegetarians have plenty of fibre from vegetables, nuts and pulses (especially beans).

Beans

Unfortunately beans take a long time to prepare because they are hard and dried. Soaking speeds up the cooking time but it is still a lengthy process. A pressure cooker will also shorten the cooking time, and beans can be cooked in quantity and stored in the freezer until needed.

To cook beans

1   Wash in cold water and remove any bad beans and stones.
2   Soak in cold water overnight. If beans are wanted in a hurry and you have forgotten to soak overnight put in a pan of cold water, bring to the boil and soak for 45–60 minutes.
3   Rinse the beans again.
4   Put in a saucepan. Just cover with water, bring to the boil and cook for the time shown in the table on page 91.

To pressure cook

1   Soaking is not necessary.
2   Rinse.
3   Put in the pressure cooker, cover with water. Put lid and 15 lb weight on. Heat until a steady hiss of steam is coming out.
4   Lower the heat until the hiss is gentle.
5   Cook for time shown in the table on page 91.

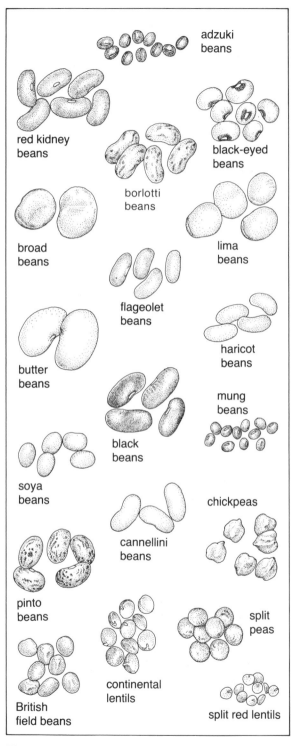

Figure 8.38   Beans, peas and lentils which provide protein and fibre in the diet

Type of bean	Cooking time in minutes	
	in a saucepan	in a pressure cooker
Adzuki	30	10
Black	60	20
Black-eyed	45	10
Borlotti	60	20
Field	30	10
Broad	90	30
Butter	75	25
Cannellini	60	20
Haricot	90	25
Kidney	60	20
Lima	60	20
Mung	30	10
Pinto	90	30
Soya	3 hours	1 hour
Dried peas	45	15
Split peas	30	10
Red split lentils	15	5

Warning

When cooking dried pulse vegetables, e.g. kidney beans, soya beans, they must be soaked for about 8 hours to soften. Red kidney beans **must** then be boiled for at least 15 minutes to destroy a natural poison (toxin) they contain. If eaten raw or partly cooked they can cause food poisoning. Pressure cooking will speed up the cooking of pulses as no soaking is then necessary.

Vegans

Vegans are strict vegetarians and will not eat or use *any* products from animals.

They have to get all their protein from plant foods and this is not easy because plant foods do not contain as much protein. Vegans need to eat a wide variety of beans, pulses, cereals and nuts.

Main meal vegetable dishes

These dishes would be suitable for lacto vegetarians.

Lentil and walnut loaf

Serve for main meal
Serve with salad, or tomato sauce (see page 113), potatoes and a fresh vegetable
Serves 4

Cook at Reg 5
190°C
Time 1 hour

Ingredients

150 g lentils
1 onion
1 teaspoon dried thyme
100 g walnuts
100 g wholemeal bread
1 tablespoon tomato purée
Parsley
1 egg
Pinch black pepper
Tomato to garnish

Method

1 Put the oven on. Grease and line a 15 × 10 cm loaf tin.
2 Cook the lentils in a pressure cooker covered with water for 10 minutes (*or* soak for a few hours and simmer in a saucepan for 40 minutes).
3 Peel and chop the onion.
4 Wash, dry and chop 1 tablespoon parsley.
5 Grind the nuts in the blender or food processor.
6 Make the bread into breadcrumbs.
7 Add the onion and thyme to the lentils and cook together for a few minutes.
8 Add the nuts, breadcrumbs, tomato purée, parsley, pepper and egg.
9 Spoon into the loaf tin and cover with a piece of greased greaseproof paper.
10 Cook until firm. Turn out and garnish with sliced tomato and parsley.

Vegetable curry or Egg curry

Serve for main meal
Serve with rice and accompaniments (see page 52)
Serves 2

Ingredients

A mixture of vegetables, e.g. carrot, cauliflower, runner beans, cooked kidney beans, tomato, celery, turnip, okra, peas (frozen vegetables may be used, but only add for the last 10 minutes)
or 2 hard boiled eggs

1 onion
1 level tablespoon wholemeal flour
$\frac{1}{2}$ teaspoon ground ginger
$\frac{1}{2}$ teaspoon turmeric
$\frac{1}{2}$ teaspoon ground cumin
$\frac{1}{2}$ teaspoon ground coriander
$\frac{1}{2}$ teaspoon garam masala (see page 52)
1 tablespoon chopped fresh coriander *or* parsley
250 ml water or vegetable stock
Squeeze of lemon juice
1 small eating apple
25 g sultanas
1 dessertspoon chutney
100 g brown rice

This makes a very mild curry. If you like it hotter add 1 cm peeled and chopped root ginger and/or half a very small seeded, chopped chilli at stage 7.

Method

1 Prepare the vegetables (wash, peel and chop into small pieces) *or* hard boil the eggs.
2 Peel and chop the onion and apple.
3 Wash and chop the parsley or coriander.
4 Toss the vegetables in the flour.
5 Mix the spices to a paste with a little water. Add the rest of the water or the vegetable stock.
6 Put the fresh vegetables in a large saucepan. Add the stock and bring to the boil stirring.
7 Add the apple, sultanas, chutney and lemon juice.
8 Simmer for 30–40 minutes until the vegetables are tender. Add any frozen vegetables for the last 10 minutes.
9 Put the rice into boiling water and boil for 35–40 minutes until it feels tender when squeezed between finger and thumb.
10 Serve the curry with the rice arranged round the curry sauce and with the accompaniments in small bowls.
11 For egg curry, slice the hard boiled eggs in half lengthwise and lay on the serving dish. Pour the curry sauce over.
12 Sprinkle with chopped coriander or parsley.

Vegetable samosas

See colour photo (page 108)

Serve for main meal, snack, buffet
Serve with tomato sauce (see page 113) mint dressing (see page 110), or salad
Makes 8

Cook at Reg 6
200°C
Time 10–15 minutes

Ingredients

For the pastry

50 g wholemeal flour
50 g white flour
2 tablespoons vegetable oil
2 tablespoons water

For the filling

500 g potatoes
1 small onion
75 g frozen peas *or* chopped runner beans
½ cm root ginger
Half a small green chilli (leave this out if you do
    not want it to be too hot)
Fresh coriander
1–2 tablespoons water
½ teaspoon ground coriander
½ teaspoon garam masala
½ teaspoon ground cumin
⅛ teaspoon cayenne pepper
1 tablespoon lemon juice

1 egg for glazing

In India samosas are eaten as a snack. You can
stuff them with meat, or any vegetables. They
are usually served with a chutney. If you cannot
get any of the ingredients above you can use
other herbs and spices, but the flavour will not
be truly Indian.

Method

1   Put the oven on. Grease a baking tray.
2   Make the pastry, mixing the oil into the
     flour with a fork.
3   Add the water a little at a time until you
     have a stiff dough.
4   Knead the dough for 5 minutes. Rub the
     outside of the dough with a little oil and put
     it in a polythene bag for about 30 minutes.

To prepare the filling

5   Scrub the potatoes and boil in their jackets
     for 20 minutes or until tender.
6   Peel and chop the onion finely.
7   Peel and chop the root ginger very finely.
     Cut off the stalk from the chilli and chop
     very finely. Wash and chop 1½ tablespoons
     coriander.
8   Dice the potatoes into 5 mm cubes.
9   Put all the filling ingredients together in a
     saucepan and cook gently together for 5
     minutes. Do not stir too much.

To make the samosas

10   Knead the pastry dough again.
11   Divide the dough into four. Shape into
      balls. Keep three covered while you work
      with the fourth.
12   Roll each ball into a 15 cm circle. Cut in half.
13   Pick up one half and shape into a cone.
      Overlap the 'seam' 5 mm and brush with
      water to seal.
14   Fill the cone with some of the filling.
15   Brush the top with water and seal.
16   Turn each samosa so that the join is
      underneath, place on a baking tray and
      brush with egg.
17   Bake until golden.

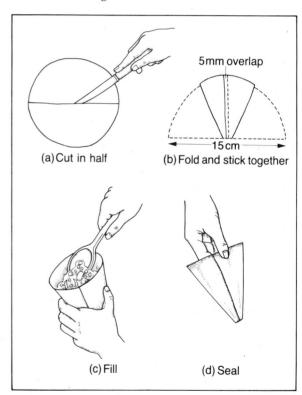

Figure 8.39   Making the samosas

Red bean moussaka

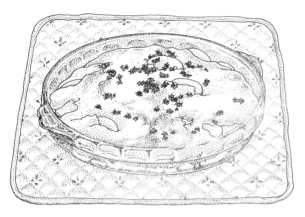

Figure 8.40

Serve for main meal
Serve with a green
vegetable or salad
Serves 4

Cook at Reg 6
200°C
Time 30–40 minutes

Ingredients

600 g potatoes
1 onion
3 tomatoes
1 tablespoon tomato purée
Shake of black pepper
½ teaspoon cinnamon
225 g canned *or* cooked kidney beans (see page 91)
1 egg
250 ml skimmed milk
25 g polyunsaturated margarine
25 g wholemeal flour
75 g firm low fat cheese
Parsley

Method

1   Put the oven on.
2   Peel the potatoes. Cut into quarters if large. Boil until just tender (about 20 minutes). Cool, then cut into thin slices.
3   Grate the cheese.
4   Peel and chop the onions and tomatoes.
5   Wash and chop the parsley.
6   Mix the tomatoes, onion, pepper, cinnamon, tomato purée and beans together, mashing the beans slightly.
7   Make a roux sauce (see page 114) using the flour, margarine and milk. Cool slightly.
8   Mix the egg into the sauce.
9   Put a layer of potato slices in a casserole dish, then a layer of bean mixture, then a layer of a sauce. Repeat this, finishing with a layer of sauce.
10 Sprinkle with cheese.
11 Bake until golden brown.
12 Sprinkle with chopped parsley.

Wholemeal pasties

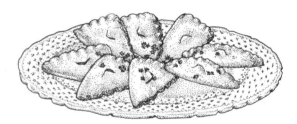

Figure 8.41

Serve for main meal,
packed meal
Serve with salad
Makes 6

Cook at Reg 6
200°C
Time 30 minutes

Ingredients

For the pastry

100 g wholemeal flour
100 g white flour
100 g polyunsaturated margarine
Water to mix

Filling (see below)

Egg to glaze

Filling

Choose from:

Tomato and cheese

1 onion, peeled and chopped
2 tomatoes, peeled and chopped
1 slice wholemeal bread, made into breadcrumbs
50 g firm low fat cheese, grated

Cheese and egg

3 eggs, hard boiled and chopped
50 g polyunsaturated margarine ⎫ Made into a
50 g wholemeal flour　　　　　 ⎬ roux sauce
250 ml skimmed milk　　　　　 ⎭ (see page 114)
50 g firm low fat cheese, grated

Mushroom

1 onion, peeled and chopped
50 g mushrooms, washed and chopped
1 level teaspoon mixed dried herbs
1 egg, hard boiled and chopped

Method

1　Put the oven on. Grease a baking tray.
2　Prepare the chosen filling, mixing all the ingredients together.
3　Put the flour for the pastry in a bowl. Rub in the fat until like fine breadcrumbs.
4　Add enough water to give a stiff dough.
5　Roll out 5 mm thick. Cut into 6 squares.
6　Divide the filling into six and place some diagonally on each piece of pastry. Do not overfill.
7　Brush the edges with water. Fold over. Seal by pressing the edges together. Flake and flute the edges (see page 62).
8　Place on the baking tray and brush with egg. Make an air hole in the top of each with a knife or by snipping with scissors.
9　Bake until golden brown.

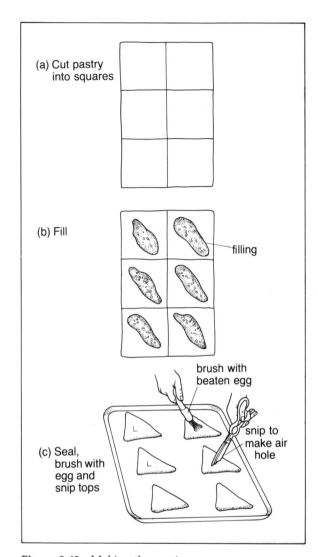

Figure 8.42　Making the pasties

Nutty Scotch eggs

The lentil and walnut loaf mixture can be used to coat hard boiled eggs for a version of Scotch eggs which have less fat than the usual sausage meat coating. They are cooked in the oven, instead of being fried in deep fat, to cut down the fat still more.

Ingredients

Lentil and walnut loaf mixture (as on page 91)
4 hard boiled eggs
A little wholemeal flour
2 eggs
Dried breadcrumbs

Method

1 Put the oven on Reg 4 or 180°C.
2 Hard boil the eggs. Cool by putting into cold water. Peel.
3 Coat the eggs in flour, then press some of the lentil and walnut mixture round the eggs, covering completely.
4 Dip in beaten egg, followed by the dried crumbs (Figure 8.43).

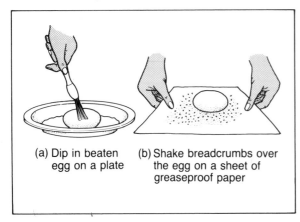

(a) Dip in beaten egg on a plate   (b) Shake breadcrumbs over the egg on a sheet of greaseproof paper

Figure 8.43

5 Place on the baking tray and cook for 15 minutes. Turn and cook 10–15 minutes more.
6 Serve with salad or tomato sauce.

Vegetable pie

Serve for main meal
Serve with green salad
Serves 3

Ingredients

400 g potatoes + a little skimmed milk
250 ml skimmed milk
25 g wholemeal flour
25 g polyunsaturated margarine
400 g mixed vegetables (e.g. peas, carrots, sweetcorn, beans)
75 g firm low fat cheese
1 tomato
Parsley

Method

1 Put a shallow casserole dish to warm.
2 Peel the potatoes. Cut into small pieces. Cook in boiling water for about 20 minutes, until tender.
3 Prepare the vegetables (large vegetables should be diced). Cook in boiling water until tender.
4 Grate the cheese.
5 Skin and slice the tomato.
6 Make a roux sauce (see page 114) using the flour, margarine and milk.
7 Stir in the cheese, saving a little for the top.
8 Mash the potatoes with milk until smooth. Pipe the potatoes round the sides and bottom of the casserole dish.
9 Brush with milk and grill until crisp.

10 Mix the vegetables into the sauce.
11 Pour into the potato case. Sprinkle with
     cheese.
12 Grill until golden brown.
13 Garnish with parsley.

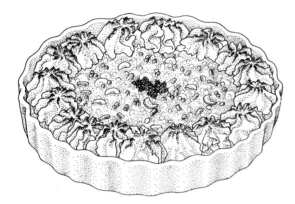

Figure 8.44

See also cheese recipes (pages 78–82)
           egg recipes (pages 85–86)
           vegetable recipes (pages 101–104)

9 Accompaniments

Vegetables

Vegetables can be eaten either as an accompaniment to a meal or as a main course. They are mostly eaten for the vitamins, minerals, protein and fibre they contain.

Nutrients in vegetables

Green vegetables, e.g. broccoli, sprouts and peppers, contain vitamin C and so do potatoes.

Vitamin A is found in dark green and orange coloured vegetables, e.g. carrots, spinach, broccoli and cabbage.

Vitamin B is found in green vegetables, peas and beans.

Fibre is found particularly in the skins of potatoes and in beans, sweetcorn and peas.

Some root vegetables also contain carbohydrate in their roots, e.g. beetroot, parsnip, potato and carrot.

Protein is found in peas, beans and sprouts.

Calcium and iron are found in many vegetables including cabbage, lentils, and spinach but the body is not able to use all of this because of the oxalic acid, or possibly other substances, they also contain. Spinach is not really the good source of iron that Popeye made it out to be.

Vegetables should be eaten fresh to save all the vitamins. Frozen vegetables are nearly as good, as they are mainly frozen straight from the fields. Canned (especially processed) and dried vegetables will have lost much of their vitamins.

Storing vegetables

Potatoes and other root vegetables should be stored in a cool dark place so they do not sprout.

Leaf vegetables lose vitamin C and water quickly so should be kept in a polythene bag in a cool place — the refrigerator salad drawer is a good place.

Vegetables should not be stored for long or their vitamins will be lost.

Table 9.1

Leaves	Fruit	Seeds/pods	Stems	Flowers	Roots	Bulbs	Tubers
Cabbage	Cucumber	Peas	Celery	Cauliflower	Carrots	Onions	Potatoes
Brussels sprouts	Tomato	Runner beans	Asparagus	Broccoli	Beetroot	Leeks	Jerusalem artichokes
Spinach	Marrow	French beans	Fennel		Swedes		Sweet potatoes
Watercress	Sweetcorn	Okra			Parsnips		Yams
Chicory	Peppers	Broad beans			Radishes		
Globe artichokes	Aubergines Courgettes	Pulses i.e. dried peas, beans. lentils			Turnips		
					Salsify		
		(see page 90)					

Cooking vegetables

To avoid losing vitamins:

1 Buy fresh and eat as soon as possible

2 Eat uncooked when possible or cook quickly for a short length of time.

3 Use only a little water (and use the left-over water for a soup, gravy or sauce).

4 Eat the vegetables as soon as they are ready and do not leave standing.

5 Shred rather than grate, or tear by hand if possible.

6 Do not add bicarbonate of soda. Vegetables will keep their colour without this if they are cooked for only a short length of time.

Different types of vegetables

Vegetables can be divided into types by where they come from on the plant (see table above).

Questions

1 Find out which ingredients are used in salads around the world. For example, where is fennel served? What is endive? How would you serve Chinese leaves?

2 Some vegetables are served stuffed to make a main meal dish out of a vegetable. Find a recipe in another book for: stuffed peppers, marrow, vine leaves.

3 You can buy some salad dressings made-up, but they may be high in kilocalories (kilojoules), salt or fat. Find a label for a bought salad dressing and list the ingredients. Write beside it the recipe you could use if you made the dressing yourself.

Cooking potatoes

Potatoes are a popular and economical vegetable, but they are often served only as chips (very fatty) or plainly boiled or mashed. There are many more interesting ways to serve potatoes and a few of them are given in the table on page 100.

Table 9.2

All potato dishes serve 4. N.B. In the first three recipes the potato skins are left on as they contain the fibre. Make sure the potatoes are scrubbed well, and cut out any bad bits particularly in old potatoes. Always leave the skins on if you can.			
Dish	**Preparation**	**Method**	**Cooking**
Rosemary potatoes 400 g potatoes 200 ml milk Dried rosemary Black pepper	Scrub and slice potatoes thinly (the food processor is good for this).	Arrange layers of potato sprinkled with rosemary and pepper in a casserole dish. Pour milk over. Cover.	Cook 1–1½ hours at Reg 6 or 200° C until tender or microwave 20–30 minutes.
Rosemary and onion potatoes As above but add 1 small onion	As above, but also peel and slice onion thinly.	Arrange onion in layers with potato, rosemary and pepper. Cover.	As above.
Saucy potatoes 400 g potatoes 25 g polyunsaturated margarine 25 g wholemeal flour 250 ml skimmed milk 75 g firm low fat cheese Pinch black pepper	Scrub and boil potatoes until tender (about 20 minutes). Slice thickly. Grate cheese. Make roux sauce with milk, flour and margarine. Stir in half the grated cheese and the pepper.	Arrange sliced potatoes in a casserole dish. Pour sauce over. Sprinkle with grated cheese.	Grill until golden brown. N.B. The potatoes for this, and the next two dishes, could be microwaved with 6 tablespoons of water (covered) for 10 minutes.
Potato galette 600 g potatoes 1 small onion ¼ teaspoon black pepper ½ teaspoon paprika Parsley 6 tablespoons skimmed milk 1 egg	Scrub, peel and boil the potatoes until tender (about 20 minutes). Wash and chop the parsley. Peel and chop the onion. Mash the potatoes and mix in the other ingredients except the paprika.	Spoon into a greased flan dish. Sprinkle pepper over.	Bake at Reg 5 or 190° C until golden brown and crisp.
Duchesse potatoes 400 g potatoes 1 egg 4 tablespoons skimmed milk	Scrub, peel and boil the potatoes until tender (about 20 minutes) Add the milk and half the beaten egg and mash. Beat with a wooden spoon until smooth.	Pipe onto a greased baking tray. whirl large star nozzle star	Cook in the oven for 5 minutes at Reg 6 or 200° C. Remove and brush with remaining beaten egg. Return to the oven and cook 8–10 minutes until golden.
Surprise potatoes See page 34			

Vegetable roundup

Here are some more interesting ways of cooking common vegetables.

All vegetable dishes serve 4.

See colour photo (page 108)

Hungarian beans

Ingredients

400 g French *or* runner beans
1 large or 2 medium onions
1 tablespoon paprika
300 g fresh *or* canned tomatoes
1 tablespoon tomato purée

Method

1   Wash the beans. Cut into 5 cm lengths.
2   Peel and chop the onion.
3   Chop the canned tomatoes *or* peel and chop the fresh tomatoes.
4   Put the tomatoes, beans, onion, paprika and tomato purée into a large saucepan.
5   Cover and cook for 15–20 minutes until tender.
6   Serve in a vegetable dish.

This dish may also be cooked in the microwave. Put the ingredients in a dish with a lid and cook for 10–15 minutes.

Stuffed tomatoes

Ingredients

8 tomatoes
Filling (see below)
3–4 slices wholemeal bread
Parsley

Fillings

Choose from:

Vegetable

Small packet frozen peas or mixed vegetables, cooked as on the packet

Sardine

Can sardines, drained and mashed

Mushroom, onion and bacon

50 g mushrooms, sliced and cooked in a little water
1 small onion, chopped and cooked in a little water
75 g bacon, chopped and grilled

Method

1   Put the oven on Reg 5 or 190° C.
2   Prepare the filling as above.
3   Wash the tomatoes.
4   Cut a slice from the rounded end (not the stalk end as they stand better this way).
5   Scoop out the tomato with a teaspoon and chop finely.
6   Mix the chopped tomato with the filling ingredients.
7   Pile the filling into the tomato cases with a teaspoon. Put the tomato slices back as lids.
8   Bake for 10–15 minutes until tender.
9   Wash and dry the parsley.
10   Toast the bread. Using a fancy cutter cut into rings large enough to sit a tomato on.
11   Place the toast circles on a flat serving dish and sit the tomatoes on top.
12   Garnish with parsley.

This dish may also be microwaved. Cook the tomatoes for 5–10 minutes. Watch them, as they cook very quickly.

Algerian carrots

Ingredients

800 g carrots
Pinch black pepper
$\frac{1}{4}$ teaspoon ground cinnamon
$\frac{1}{2}$ teaspoon cumin seeds
$\frac{1}{2}$ teaspoon dried thyme
1 bayleaf
1 teaspoon lemon juice
Parsley

Method

1   Scrub, peel and slice the carrots into rings.
2   Just cover with water and add the other ingredients, except the lemon juice and parsley.
3   Cook for about 20 minutes until tender.
4   Wash, dry and chop the parsley.
5   Strain. Remove the bayleaf. Sprinkle with lemon juice.
6   Serve in a vegetable dish with chopped parsley sprinkled down the middle.

This dish may also be cooked in the microwave. Cook in a covered dish adding 100 ml water, for 10–12 minutes.

Conservative carrots

Conservative carrots are a good way of cooking carrots if you have other dishes cooking in the oven. The carrots can be cooked alongside the meat or other main dish, saving fuel.

Put the carrots in a casserole dish which has a lid. Add the flavouring ingredients which are the same as for Algerian carrots. Just cover with water and cook for 1–2 hours below or beside whatever is cooking in the oven. Drain, remove bayleaf, sprinkle with lemon juice and serve in a clean vegetable dish.

Cauliflower with tomatoes and cheese

Ingredients

1 large cauliflower
6 tomatoes
Pinch black pepper
50 g wholemeal bread
50 g firm low fat cheese

Method

1   Put the oven on Reg 5 or 190° C.
2   Wash the cauliflower. Break into small pieces.
3   Cook in a pan of water for 12–15 minutes until tender.
4   Skin and slice the tomatoes. Grate the cheese.
5   Make breadcrumbs with the bread.
6   Mix the breadcrumbs, cheese and pepper together.
7   Drain the cauliflower. Place in an ovenproof vegetable dish.
8   Arrange the sliced tomatoes on top of the cauliflower. Sprinkle with the bread and cheese mixture.
9   Bake for about 30 minutes until the top is golden.

This vegetable dish does not need any attention at the last minute and is useful if you are serving other dishes which do.

Peas with bacon and onion

Ingredients

4 slices lean bacon
1 small onion
Medium sized packet of frozen peas
Pinch black pepper

Method

1 Remove any fat from the bacon. Grill.
2 Peel and chop the onion. Cook in a little water until tender.
3 Add the peas and enough water to just cover. Cook for the time suggested on the packet.
4 Chop the bacon.
5 Drain the peas. Mix the bacon and pepper in and serve in a vegetable dish.

Lentil and mushroom slice

Ingredients

175 g split red lentils
350 ml water + half a stock cube
1 large onion
175 g mushrooms
100 g firm low fat cheese
1 egg
Black pepper
Parsley

Method

1 Put the oven on Reg 5 or 190° C. Grease a Swiss roll tin or similar shaped casserole.
2 Put the lentils in a saucepan with the stock cube and water. Bring to the boil and simmer until soft and all the liquid has disappeared.
3 Peel and chop the onion finely.
4 Wash and slice the mushrooms.
5 Grate the cheese.
6 Wash, dry and chop 1 tablespoon parsley.
7 Add the mushrooms and onions to the lentils, together with the parsley, a pinch of black pepper, the cheese and egg.
8 Spread the mixture in the greased tin.
9 Bake for 35 minutes until set and golden brown.

10 Cut into slices and serve with tomato sauce (see page 113).

This dish may also be served for a main meal. Serve with potatoes and fresh green vegetables.

Cabbage and carrots

Ingredients

300 g cabbage
300 g carrots
1 small green chilli (leave this out if you do not like hot foods)
1 tablespoon lemon juice
Parsley

Method

A food processor makes preparing the vegetables for this recipe easy.

1 Cut the cabbage in half, then into quarters. Cut out the stem in the middle.
2 Shred finely.
3 Scrub and peel the carrots. Grate.
4 Wash and chop the chilli very finely. Wash, dry and chop 1 tablespoon parsley.
5 Heat a pan containing 5 cm water to boiling. Add the carrots, cabbage and chilli.
6 Turn the heat down until the vegetables are just simmering and cook for 5 minutes or until the vegetables are just cooked (still crisp).
7 Drain. Add the lemon juice and parsley.
8 Serve in a vegetable dish.

This dish can also be cooked in the microwave. Add 10 tablespoons of water to the vegetables and cook in a covered dish for 10 minutes.

Carrots with bacon

Ingredients

400 g carrots
200 g lean bacon
½ teaspoon grated nutmeg
Pinch black pepper
50 g firm low fat cheese
Parsley

Method

1 Scrub, peel and slice the carrots into rings.
2 Cook, just covered with water, for 15–20 minutes until tender. Drain.
3 Cut the fat off the bacon. Grill. Chop into small pieces.
4 Grate the cheese finely. Wash and dry the parsley.
5 Mix the carrots, bacon, nutmeg and pepper together. Put into an ovenproof vegetable dish or small individual dishes.
6 Sprinkle with grated cheese. Grill until golden. Garnish with parsley.

Salads

Salads are usually made from a mixture of fresh or cooked vegetables, or fruits. They can be served as:
(a) an accompaniment to a meal instead of or as well as vegetables;
(b) a complete main course with meat, fish, cheese, eggs or poultry;
(c) a starter;
(d) in sandwich fillings.

Nutrients in salads

Like vegetables, salads provide vitamins, particularly vitamin C, minerals and fibre. As vitamins and minerals can be easily lost, salad foods should be eaten soon after buying, prepared just before eating and shredded rather than grated. Except when oily dressings are added salads are low in kilocalories (kilojoules).

Below are some salad ingredients and the main nutrients they provide.

Lettuce	
Cucumber	(mainly water)
Watercress	
Mustard and cress	Calcium and vitamin A
Onion, spring onions	Calcium
Tomato	Vitamins A and C and calcium
Radish	Vitamin C
Celery	A little calcium (mainly water)
Peppers	Vitamin C
Carrot	Vitamin A and calcium
Cabbage	Vitamin C and calcium
Cauliflower	Vitamin C and calcium
Beetroot	Calcium
Potato	Vitamin C
Beans (kidney, runner, French etc.)	Fibre
Apple	A little vitamin C (gives a crunchy texture)
Banana	Vitamins A and C and calcium
Grapes	(added mainly for colour)
Orange	Vitamin C
Pineapple	Vitamin C and calcium
Dried fruits (sultanas, raisins etc.)	Calcium and iron
Nuts (peanuts, walnuts etc.)	Fibre; peanuts provide vitamin E

Salad dressings

Salad dressings such as French dressing or mayonnaise are often served with salad to add flavour and moisture and to help in chewing and digestion. They should be put on at the last minute otherwise they make the salad ingredients go soft.

Garnishes

Salad ingredients are colourful and can be

arranged to look attractive. Extra colour or nutrients may be added by garnishing with:

    finely grated cheese
    sieved hard boiled egg
    chopped nuts
    chopped fresh herbs

Salads to serve for accompaniment

The following salads could be served as an accompaniment.
All recipes are for 4 portions.

Wholemeal pasta salad

See colour photo (page 109)

Ingredients

175 g wholemeal pasta shells
50 g sweetcorn
1 small green pepper
1 small red pepper
1 small onion
50 g mushrooms
French dressing (see page 111) *or* piquant tomato
    dressing (see page 110)

This may be made into a main meal salad by adding prawn, chicken or hard boiled egg.

Method

1 Cook the pasta in boiling water until tender (about 15–20 minutes).
2 Wash, deseed and chop the peppers.
3 Peel and chop the onion.
4 Wash and slice the mushrooms.
5 Mix all the salad ingredients together. Pile into a bowl.
6 Make the dressing. Add just enough to moisten.

Rice and almond salad

Ingredients

125 g brown long grain rice
2 rings canned or fresh pineapple
1 green pepper
4–6 spring onions
2 tablespoons raisins
25–50 g almonds
2–3 tablespoons French dressing (see page 111)

Method

1 Boil the rice for 35–40 minutes until tender. Drain. Spread over a flat dish to cool.
2 Make the French dressing.
3 Cut the pineapple into small pieces.
4 Wash the pepper. Cut off the top and remove the seeds and pith. Chop.
5 Wash and finely chop the spring onions.
6 Mix the rice, raisins, pineapple, onion and pepper together.
7 Toast the almonds by spreading on a sheet of kitchen foil and placing under the grill until golden. *Watch them* — they toast quickly.
8 Mix the dressing into the salad. Put into a shallow dish and sprinkle the almonds on top.

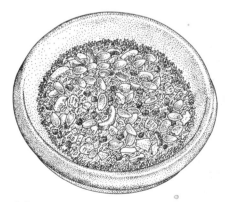

Figure 9.2

Apple and raisin coleslaw

See colour photo (page 109)

Ingredients

225 g cabbage.
3 dessert apples
25–50 g raisins
1 lemon
2 tablespoons natural yogurt
Parsley

Method

1 Remove damaged leaves from the cabbage. Cut into quarters. Remove the stalk. Shred finely.
2 Scrub the lemon. Grate half the rind and squeeze out the juice from half the lemon.
3 Wash, drain and chop 1 tablespoon parsley.
4 Mix the yogurt, lemon rind and juice and parsley together.
5 Wash the apples. Cut into quarters and remove the cores. Cut in fine slices.
6 Mix the cabbage, raisins, and yogurt dressing together.
7 Serve in a shallow dish.

Fruity salad

Ingredients

1 orange
1 red-skinned apple
150 g cabbage
25 g sultanas
A little French dressing (see page 111)

Method

1 Make the French dressing.
2 Peel the orange and cut into segments (see page 44).

3 Remove damaged leaves from the cabbage. Cut into quarters. Remove the stalk. Shred finely.
4 Wash the apple. Cut into quarters and remove the core Cut into thin slices.
5 Mix the cabbage, apple, orange and sultanas, together.
6 Add just enough of the dressing to coat the vegetables and prevent the apple from going brown.

Mexican bean salad

Ingredients

225 g canned red kidney beans *or* 200 g dried kidney beans pressure cooked for 15 minutes and cooled
1 small cauliflower
1 small green pepper
2 sticks celery
2 spring onions
Parsley
French dressing (see page 111) *or* piquant tomato dressing (see page 110)

Method

1 Make the French dressing *or* piquant tomato dressing.
2 Wash and dry the cauliflower. Break into small pieces.
3 Wash and chop the pepper. Cut off the top. Remove the seeds and pith.
4 Wash the celery. Cut into fine slices.
5 Wash and chop the onions.
6 Wash, dry and chop the parsley.
7 Drain the kidney beans.
8 Mix all the salad ingredients together.
9 Add enough dressing to coat well.
10 Serve in a salad dish.

Potato salad

Ingredients

350 g new potatoes
Yogurt dressing (see page 111)
1–2 spring onions *or* some chives *or* parsley
Watercress *or* tomato to garnish

Method

1 Scrub potatoes. Cook in the skins in boiling water until tender (about 20 minutes).
2 Drain. Cool. Cut into 5 mm cubes.
3 Wash, dry and chop the spring onions, parsley or chives. Wash and dry the watercress or tomato.
4 Make the dressing.
5 Mix the onions, parsley or chives with the potatoes.
6 Add enough dressing to coat well.
7 Garnish with sprigs of watercress or slices of tomato.

Main meal salads

These salads contain some protein foods and could form a main course.

All recipes serve 4.

Salad Niçoise

Ingredients

100 g French *or* runner beans
1 crunchy lettuce
1 small onion *or* a few spring onions
1 green pepper
3 tomatoes
French dressing (see page 111)
75 g canned tuna in brine
1 egg

Method

1 Wash the beans and cut into 2 cm lengths. Cook in boiling water until tender (about 15–20 minutes). Drain and cool.
2 Hard boil the egg. Cool.
3 Wash, dry and tear the lettuce into small pieces.
4 Peel and chop the onion finely.
5 Wash the pepper. Cut the top off. Remove the seeds and pith. Slice finely into rings.
6 Wash the tomatoes. Cut into quarters.
7 Make the French dressing.
8 Drain the tuna. Wipe off any excess brine with kitchen paper.
9 Cut the egg into quarters.
10 Mix all the salad ingredients together.
11 Just before serving add enough French dressing to moisten, and toss well.

This is a French salad and is traditionally served with olives on top and anchovies in place of the tuna. You can leave out the tuna and egg and serve this as a side salad.

Winter cheese salad

Ingredients

200 g firm low fat cheese *or* cottage cheese
5 tablespoons yogurt dressing (see page 111)
2 carrots
4 sticks celery
A few grapes
50 g peanuts

Method

1 Make the dressing.
2 Wash the celery. Chop finely.
3 Scrub and peel the carrots. Grate.
4 Wash the grapes and remove the seeds.
5 Cut firm cheese into 1 cm cubes.
6 Mix the salad ingredients together with enough dressing to moisten.
7 Spread on a plate. Pile cheese in the centre.

This is a good salad to make in the winter when fresh salad vegetables may be expensive.

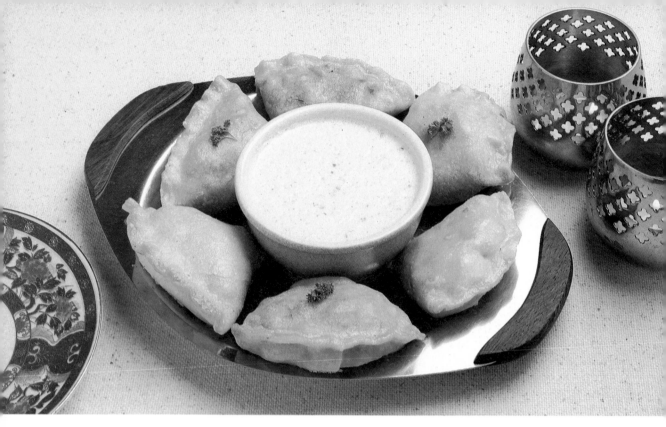

Vegetable samosas with mint dressing (page 92) ▲

Hungarian beans, Cabbage and carrots, Algerian carrots, Stuffed tomatoes (pages 101–103) ▼

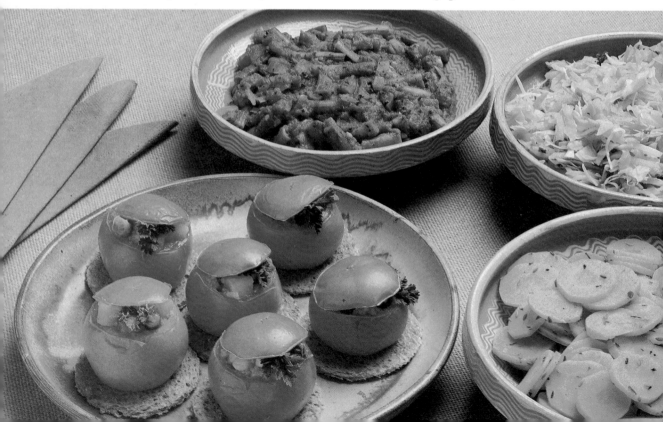

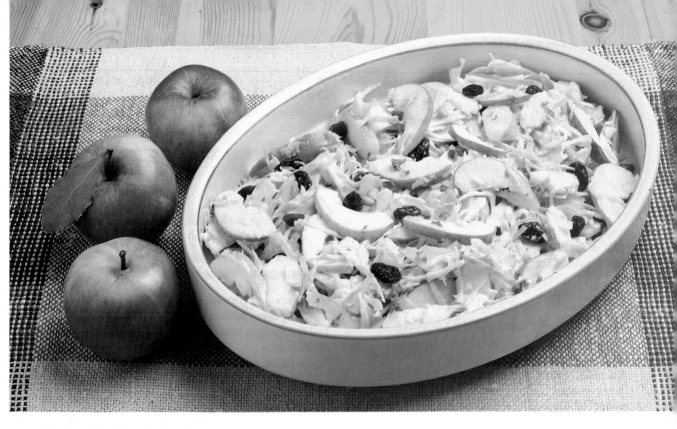

Apple and raisin coleslaw (page 106) ▲

Wholemeal pasta salad (page 105) ▼

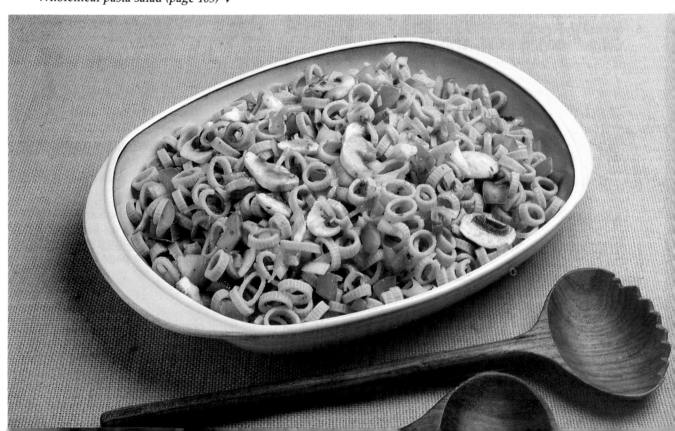

Apple and date slices

Serve for pudding,
packed meal, buffet,
tea
Serve with custard (if hot)
Serves 4

Cook at Reg 6
200°C
Time 40–45 minutes

Ingredients

For the pastry

100 g wholemeal flour
100 g white flour
75 g polyunsaturated margarine
Water to mix

For the filling

350 g cooking apples
100 g dates
50 g walnuts
50 g demerara sugar

For the topping

225 g wholemeal flour
100 g polyunsaturated margarine
25 g demerara sugar
1 teaspoon cinnamon

Method

1 Make the shortcrust pastry (see page 128).
2 Roll out and line a Swiss roll tin. Flute the edges.
3 Wash, peel, core and chop and chop the apples. Chop the dates and walnuts. Mix the fruit and nuts with sugar and spread over the pastry.
4 Make the topping by rubbing the margarine into the flour. Stir in the sugar and cinnamon. Sprinkle over the filling.
5 Bake 40–45 minutes until golden.
6 Cool slightly. Cut into slices.
7 Serve hot with custard, or allow to go cold.

Fruit crumble

Serve for pudding
Serve with custard
Serves 4

Cook at Reg 6
200°C
Time 30–35 minutes

Ingredients

600 g cooking apples or other fruit
50 g sugar

For the crumble topping

50 g mixed chopped nuts
50 g porridge oats
100 g wholemeal flour
30 g polyunsaturated margarine
25 g demerara sugar

Method

1 Put the oven on. Grease a shallow casserole dish.
2 Put the nuts, oats, flour, margarine and demerara sugar in a mixing bowl.
3 Rub the fat into the flour until the mixture looks like fine breadcrumbs.
4 Wash, peel, core and slice the apples.
5 Put in the casserole dish in layers with sugar.
6 Spread the crumble mixture over.
7 Bake for 30–35 minutes until golden brown.
8 Serve with custard.

This crumble topping has less fat than usual and extra fibre.

Baked stuffed apples

Serve for pudding
Serve with custard
Serves 2

Cook at Reg 5 190°C
Time 1 hour *or*
Microwave 3–4 minutes

Ingredients

2 large cooking apples
1 tablespoon golden syrup

For the filling

A mixture of dried fruits (e.g. sultanas, raisins, currants, apricots) *or* mincemeat

Method

1 Put the oven on.
2 Put the syrup with 150 ml water in a casserole dish.
3 Wash the apples. Core. Score round the middle with the point of a knife.
4 Place the apples in the dish and fill with chosen filling.
5 Bake until the apples feel tender when a knife is pushed in *or* microwave for about 4 minutes until tender.

Baked banana tart

Serve for pudding	Cook at Reg 5
Serve with custard	190°C
Serves 4	Time 45 minutes

Ingredients

For the pastry

75 g wholemeal flour
50 g white flour
60 g polyunsaturated margarine
Water to mix

For the filling

50 g wholemeal flour
1 rounded teaspoon baking powder
50 g caster sugar
50 g polyunsaturated margarine

1 egg
Few drops almond essence
2 bananas
2 tablespoons jam

Icing sugar

Method

1 Put the oven on.
2 Make shortcrust pastry by rubbing the fat into the flour until like fine breadcrumbs.
3 Add enough water to make a stiff dough, mixing with a knife.
4 Roll out to fit a 20 cm flan ring. Place the flan ring on a baking tray. Line the flan ring with pastry.
5 Spread the jam in the bottom of the flan case.
6 Make a creamed mixture (see page 140) with the margarine, sugar, egg, almond essence and flour.
7 Peel and slice the bananas. Spread the slices over the flan case.
8 Spoon the cake mixture over.
9 Bake until the cake is springy when touched.
10 Sprinkle very lightly with icing sugar.

Raspberry shortbread pie

Serve for pudding	Cook at Reg 5
Serve with custard	190°C
Serves 4	Time 25–30 minutes

Ingredients

125 g wholemeal flour
100 g white flour
125 g polyunsaturated margarine
100 g demerara sugar
200 g raspberries (*or* use blackcurrants, strawberries, gooseberries) fresh or frozen

Method

1 Put the oven on. Grease a flan ring and baking tray.
2 Rub the fat into the flour and sugar until like fine breadcrumbs.
3 Put one third of the mixture on one side and save.
4 Continue rubbing in the rest of the mixture until it forms a stiff paste.
5 Press the paste round the bottom and sides of the flan ring.
6 Place the fruit on top.
7 Sprinkle with the rest of the crumble.
8 Bake until golden brown

Sweets

When making cold sweets try to use fresh fruits and include wholemeal flour or cereals for fibre. If using canned fruit use the unsweetened sort.

Many cold sweets are made up of a foam of egg whites and fruit. To set this, **gelatine** is often used. Gelatine comes from the skin, bones and tendons of cattle which have been slaughtered for meat. It is also used for setting savoury dishes, such as fish moulds, for souffles and Turkish delight. These dishes would, therefore, not be suitable for vegetarians.

Gelatine is tasteless and has no smell. When it is mixed with water it makes a gel and if this is warmed it becomes liquid. When cooled it sets. The best way to melt gelatine is to put it, with a little water, in a small basin in a pan of water and warm gently (or dissolve in a basin in the microwave for 1–2 minutes).

Using gelatine to make sweets is better than using a commercial jelly which contains a lot of sugar and added colourings.

Arrowroot, eggs and cornflour are also used to set sweets.

Many cold sweets have a base of pastry, cake or biscuit. These will have more fat than those made just from fruit or milk. Whisked sponges, though, contain little fat.

Fruit flan (sponge base)

Serve for sweet, buffet	Cook at Reg 4 180°C
Serves 4–6	Time 20–25 minutes

Ingredients

2 eggs
25 g wholemeal flour
25 g white flour
50 g caster sugar
Fresh or canned fruit in unsweetened juice
1 rounded teaspoon arrowroot *or* 2 tablespoons apricot jam or redcurrant jelly

Method

1 Put the oven on. Grease and line the base of a flan tin.
2 Make the flan case by the whisked method (see page 131).
3 Cook 20–25 minutes until firm and golden. Cool.
4 Drain fruit *or* prepare fresh fruit and place in flan case.
5 *For arrowroot glaze* (using juice from canned fruit). Put the arrowroot in a saucepan. Gradually stir in 150 ml of fruit juice (add water if there is not enough fruit juice). Bring to the boil stirring all the time. Boil until the glaze clears. Pour over the fruit.
    For jam glaze.   Place the jam with 1 tablespoon water in a small saucepan and heat gently. Sieve to remove lumps. Pour over the fruit.

The edges of a sponge flan may be decorated before filling by making a jam glaze as above and brushing it round the sides, then rolling in chopped nuts or coconut.

Mandarin flan whip

Serve for sweet,
buffet
Serves 4–6

Cook at Reg 4
180°C
Time 20–25 minutes

Ingredients

25 wholemeal flour
25 g white flour
1 dessertspoon cocoa
2 eggs
50 g caster sugar

For the orange cream filling

3 rounded teaspoons gelatine
Small can evaporated milk
Small can mandarin oranges in unsweetened juice

Method

1 Put the oven on. Grease and line the base of a flan tin.
2 Sieve the cocoa. Make the flan case by the whisked method (see page 141) adding the cocoa with the flour.
3 Cook until firm and golden.
4 Measure 150 ml of fruit juice. Dissolve the gelatine in a little of the juice, then add the rest.
5 Chop up half the oranges. Put in the liquidiser with the milk and gelatine and liquidise until smooth.
6 Allow to partly set, then pour into the flan case.
7 When set decorate with remaining oranges.

Cheesecake

Serve for sweet, buffet
Serves 4–6

Ingredients

100 g digestive biscuits
25 g polyunsaturated margarine
200 g cottage cheese
75 g caster sugar
3 level tablespoons dried skimmed milk
1 lemon
3 level teaspoons gelatine
Fresh fruit, e.g. grapes, bananas, kiwi fruit

This cheesecake has no cream in it and uses cottage rather than cream cheese so it is lower in fat than most cheesecakes.

Method

1 Grease a flan dish or loose bottomed cake tin.
2 Crush the biscuits by placing between two sheets of greaseproof paper and pressing with a rolling pin or liquidise or use the food processor.
3 Melt the margarine. Stir in the biscuit crumbs. Press into the flan case.
4 Place the cottage cheese in the liquidiser or food processor (or sieve into a bowl). Add the sugar and dried milk.
5 Scrub the lemon. Grate half the rind and squeeze out half the juice.
6 Place the juice in a small basin with the gelatine. Put the basin in a pan of water and dissolve gently.
7 Add 125 ml water and the lemon rind. Add the gelatine to the cottage cheese and liquidise.
8 Pour over biscuit mixture. Set in the refrigerator.
9 When set decorate with fresh fruit. Toss the fruit in lemon juice first if it is likely to go brown.

Fruit fool

Serve for sweet
Serves 4

Ingredients

400 g fruit (choose fruit with strong colour and
    flavour, e.g. gooseberries, blackcurrant)
Sugar to taste (omit if possible)

For the custard

250 ml skimmed milk
1 heaped tablespoon custard powder
1 tablespoon sugar
Cherries, angelica to decorate

Method

1   Prepare the fruit. Cook. Liquidise.
2   Make thick custard. Cool.
3   Mix the ingredients together.
4   Taste and sweeten if necessary.
5   Pour into individual dishes and decorate with
    cherries and angelica.

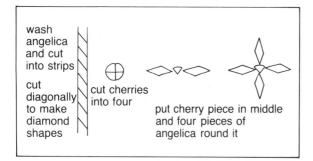

Figure 10.2   Making the decorations

Strawberry fluff

Serve for sweet, buffet
Serves 4

Ingredients

200 g fresh or frozen strawberries (*or* use other
    fresh fruit)
Small carton natural yogurt
2 level teaspoons gelatine
1 egg white
Sugar to taste (omit if possible)

Method

1   Wash the strawberries. Keep four for
    decoration. Remove stalks from the rest.
    Sieve, liquidise or purée in a food processor.
2   Add yogurt and mix well.
3   Place 4 tablespoons water with the gelatine
    in a small basin. Place the basin in a pan of
    water and stir the gelatine until it dissolves.
4   Stir into the strawberry mixture.
5   Separate the egg. Whisk the egg white until
    stiff but not dry.
6   Fold the egg white into the strawberry
    mixture. Taste and sweeten if necessary.
7   Pour into individual dishes.
8   Decorate with strawberries.

Fresh fruit salad

Serve for sweet, buffet

Ingredients

Mixture of fruit, e.g. apple, pear, banana,
    grapes, oranges, melon, plum
Lemon juice
2 oranges

Method

1 Scrub the 2 oranges and grate the rind finely.
2 Squeeze the juice from the oranges and place in a fruit bowl.
3 Prepare the fruit cutting it all to the same size. Leave bananas, apples and any other fruits which could go brown until last and sprinkle with lemon juice as they are cut.
4 Place in the bowl with the juice. If needed, 2–4 tablespoons water may be added to make the fruit more moist.

Sunflower shortcake

Serve for sweet, buffet
Serves 6

Cook at Reg 5
190°C
Time 25–30 minutes

Ingredients

75 g wholemeal flour
75 g white flour
100 g polyunsaturated margarine
50 g caster sugar
Small can mandarin oranges in unsweetened juice
1 rounded teaspoon arrowroot
Cherries to decorate

Method

1 Put the oven on. Grease a baking tray and a 20 cm flan ring.
2 Put the margarine, flour and sugar into a mixing bowl and rub together with finger tips until like breadcrumbs.
3 Pour into the flan ring and press down with a palette knife.
4 Cook until pale golden. Cool. (N.B The shortbread will not be firm until cold.)
5 Drain the fruit. Arrange on the shortbread.
6 Make the juice up to 150 ml with water.
7 Measure the arrowroot into a saucepan. Gradually mix in the fruit juice stirring all the time.

8 Bring to the boil, stirring.
9 Brush the arrowroot glaze over the fruit.
10 Decorate with a few pieces of cherry.

Apple snow

Serve for sweet
Serves 4

Ingredients

400 g cooking apples
2 tablespoons water
4 slices Swiss roll or 2 trifle sponges sandwiched together with a little jam
1 egg white
1 dessertspoon gelatine
Cherry and angelica to decorate
Sugar to taste

Method

1 Wash, peel, core and slice the apples.
2 Place with water in a saucepan and cook gently until tender (or microwave 10 minutes).
3 Place Swiss roll slices, or half trifle sponges, in the bottom of small individual dishes.
4 Sieve or liquidise the apples. Taste and sweeten if necessary.
5 Whisk the egg white until you can turn the bowl upside down without it falling out.
6 Put the gelatine in a small basin with 1 tablespoon cold water and 2 tablespoons of hot water. Stand in a pan of water and heat gently until dissolved.
7 Stir the egg white into the apple. Add the gelatine and fold together carefully.
8 Pour over the sponges.
9 Decorate as above.

11 Drinks (Beverages)

Why we need drinks

It is important to include a drink with every meal to help digestion. Liquids are also needed to replace the liquid lost every day in normal body functions. Alcoholic drinks do not help, because they cause the body to lose water (they are dehydrating) Adults should drink about 1½ litres of non-alcoholic liquid a day, children 1 litre.

Fruity drinks can provide vitamin C and milk drinks protein and calcium. Flavoured milk drinks are a good way to get young children to take milk. Coca cola and other fizzy drinks are loaded with sugar and should be avoided as they are not good for the teeth and contain only calories without any other nutrients.

Tea or coffee are often served with or after meals. They contain a stimulant called **caffeine** which can cause blood pressure to rise. Avoid drinking too many drinks containing caffeine and do not give to young children. Drinks containing stimulants like caffeine can become addictive (you cannot give them up).

Questions

1 Skimmed milk is a good way to get calcium. It is very digestible for people who have been unwell or for young children. Not everyone likes the taste of milk, though. Can you think of other flavourings for milk besides those in this book? Try not to add too much sugar.

Recipes for drinks

For orange and lemon drinks see page 27.

Mixed fruit juice

Serves 2

Ingredients

1 orange
1 grapefruit
150 ml pineapple juice

Method

1 Squeeze the juice from the orange and grapefruit.
2 Mix with pineapple juice.
3 Chill in the refrigerator.
4 Serve with a slice of orange or lemon, or mint leaves.

Frosting the glasses

For special occasions you might like to frost the glasses:
Lightly beat the white of an egg and pour onto a plate.
Put some caster sugar on a plate and spread thinly.
Take each glass and press first in the egg, then the sugar.
Leave to dry.

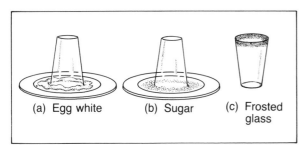

(a) Egg white   (b) Sugar   (c) Frosted glass

Figure 11.1   Frosting glasses

Banana milk shake

Serves 2

Ingredients

1 medium sized banana
600 ml skimmed milk
Powdered nutmeg

Method

1 Mash the banana well.
2 Whisk in the milk, *or* liquidise the banana and milk together.
3 Pour into a jug and sprinkle the top lightly with nutmeg.
4 Chill.

Egg flip

Serves 1

Ingredients

1 egg
150 ml skimmed milk
½ teaspoon sugar *or* 1 teaspoon glucose
1 teaspoon brandy (if allowed)

This drink is good for invalids as the egg provides extra protein.

Method

1 Separate the yolk from the white of the egg. Whisk the white until frothy.
2 Heat the milk until it steams. Beat in the yolk.
3 Fold in the white.
4 Add the brandy and sugar.
5 Pour into a glass and serve.

Strawberry flip

Serves 2

Ingredients

Small carton strawberry yogurt
250 ml skimmed milk
Whole strawberry to decorate (if in season)

Method

1 Whisk the yogurt and milk well together.
2 Pour into glasses or a jug.
3 Chill. Decorate with fresh strawberry if possible.

Cider cup

Serves 4

Ingredients

500 ml cider
250 ml soda water
150 ml orange juice
150 ml lemon squash concentrate
150 ml ginger ale
Cucumber slices to decorate

Method

1   Mix all the ingredients together, except cucumber.
2   Chill.
3   Slice cucumber thinly and float slices on top.

You might like to make this drink in larger quantities for a party.

Coffee

Jug method

Serves 2–3

Ingredients

2 rounded tablespoons ground coffee
250 ml water
250 ml skimmed milk
Brown sugar to taste

Method

1   Warm two jugs, one for the coffee and one for the milk.
2   Boil the water.
3   Put the coffee in one jug and pour the boiling water over.

4   Leave in a warm place to brew.
5   Heat the milk. *Do not* boil.
6   Put the milk into the other warmed jug.
7   Strain the coffee into cups.
8   Serve with a bowl of brown sugar.

Percolator method

Serves 2–3

Ingredients

500 ml water
4 level tablespoons ground coffee

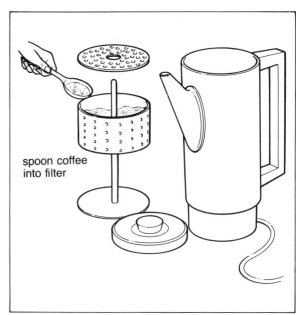

spoon coffee into filter

Figure 11.2   Coffee percolator

Method

1   Put the coffee into the perforated holder. Do not fill more than half full or it may overflow.
2   Put the water in the pot, then put the holder back in.
3   Put the lid on and put the pot on a gas or electric ring (or plug in if you are using an electric percolator).
4   Heat gently until you can see or hear the coffee beating against the lid.

5 Percolate for about 10 minutes, until the coffee looks a rich brown colour.
6 Remove the coffee holder.
7 Serve with milk and sugar, as above.

Filter method

Ingredients

1 measure of coffee per person
1 cup of water per person

Method

1 Measure the required number of cups of water into the water holder of the filter. There is usually a measure on the jug or the holder.
2 Place a filter paper in the filter holder. Measure into this one measure of coffee per cup. A measuring spoon is usually provided for this.
3 Switch on.

4 The coffee will be ready when all the water has bubbled through the coffee into the second jug.
5 Serve with milk and sugar, as above.

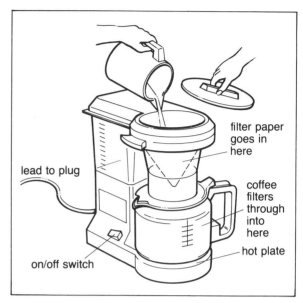

Figure 11.3   Filter method

12 Pastries

Types of pastry

Pastry is made from fat and flour. By using wholemeal flour we can add fibre to all pastries. The amount and type of fat used and the way it is mixed gives the different types:

Shortcrust pastry — half as much fat as flour
suet pastry — half as much fat as flour
flaky or rough puff pastry — two-thirds to three-quarters as much fat as flour
choux pastry — almost as much fat as flour

Suet pastry contains saturated fat which can lead to a build-up of cholesterol in the arteries. Lard and margarine can be used for shortcrust, flaky and rough puff pastry, but using all polyunsaturated margarine gives a good, slightly softer pastry.

Shortcrust pastry with wholemeal flour and polyunsaturated margarine is the best of the pastries nutritionally. Using the pastry just on the top or the bottom of a dish rather than both can also cut down on fat. The fat in **shortcrust** pastry can be reduced down to one-quarter fat to flour if a level teaspoon of baking powder is added to lighten the pastry. This does give a dryer result and may not be to everyone's taste.

Flaky and rough puff pastries are best saved only for special treats because of their high fat content.

Questions

1 List six pastry dishes. How could you cut down the amount of fat in these recipes? (For example, for an apple pie you could use pastry only on the bottom and make an apple flan, or you could make baked apples and cut down the fat still further.)

Basic pastry recipes

N.B. All pastries should be kept cool when making. Use ice cold water, rinse hands in cold water before handling and mix with a metal blade. Make as quickly as possible. Warmth softens the fat and can make the pastry oily. On a hot day place pastry in the fridge for a while before using.

Shortcrust pastry

Cook at Reg 6
200°C
Time 20–30 minutes

Ingredients

100 g wholemeal flour
100 g white flour
100 g polyunsaturated margarine
5 teaspoons water to every 100 g flour

Method (Rubbed-in method)

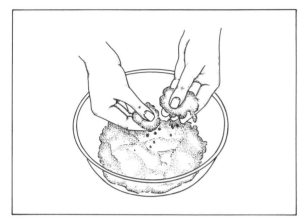

Figure 12.1 Rubbing in — lift the hands above the bowl

1 Rub margarine into flour with finger tips until the mixture is like fine breadcrumbs.
2 Add water a teaspoon at a time, mixing until the mixture starts to form large lumps.
3 Press mixture together. It should be a stiff dough.
4 Roll out 4 mm thick.
5 Use for pies, flans, tarts etc.

Cheese pastry

Add 50–75 g firm low fat cheese, grated, and a pinch of cayenne pepper to 200 g flour. Beaten egg may be used instead of water to mix.

One-stage shortcrust pastry

Ingredients

125 g wholemeal flour
100 g white flour
150 g polyunsaturated margarine
50 ml water (10 teaspoonsful)

Method

1 Put margarine, water and one-third of the flour into a mixing bowl.
2 Mix with a fork for half a minute.
3 Add the rest of the flour and mix to a firm dough.
4 Knead until smooth.

This method of making pastry is quicker, but the ingredients must be measured and handled carefully.

Rough puff pastry

Cook at Reg 7
    220°C
Time 25–30 minutes

Ingredients

100 g strong wholemeal flour
100 g strong white flour
150 g polyunsaturated margarine
1 teaspoon lemon juice
20 ml (1 tablespoon) water to each 25 g flour

Method

1 Cut the fat into walnut sized pieces.
2 Add the fat and lemon juice to the flour.
3 Adding the water 1 tablespoon at a time mix with a palette knife until there is a soft elastic dough.
4 Roll out to an oblong three times as long as it is wide. Mark into thirds as for flaky pastry (overleaf).
5 Fold the top third to the middle and the bottom third up. Seal the edges by pressing together with a rolling pin.
6 Put in the refrigerator for 5 minutes. Give a quarter turn.
7 Repeat three more times. If the dough becomes sticky put it in the refrigerator for 10 minutes.
8 Use as for flaky pastry.

Flaky pastry

Cook at Reg 7
220° C
Time 25–30 minutes

Ingredients

100 g strong wholemeal flour
100 g strong white flour
150 g polyunsaturated margarine
1 teaspoon lemon juice
20 ml (1 tablespoon) water to each 25 g flour

Method

1　Divide the margarine into four portions.
2　Add one of the portions to the flour and rub together.
3　Add the lemon juice, and mixing with a palette knife add the water 1 tablespoon at a time until there is a soft elastic dough. The lemon juice softens the gluten — the protein part of the flour — and makes a more elastic dough.
4　Roll to a rectangle three times as long as it is wide. Mark into thirds.

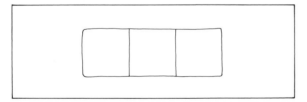

5　Using one portion of the fat, spread the fat in small blobs over the top two-thirds of the rectangle.

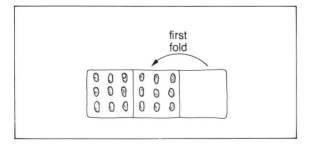

6　Fold the bottom to the middle, and the top down.

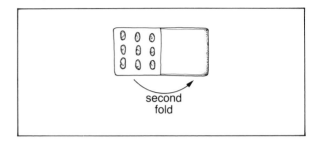

7　Seal the edges by pressing together with a rolling pin and place in the refrigerator for 5 minutes.

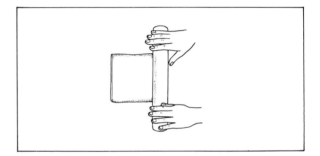

8　Turn the pastry one quarter turn.

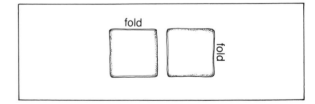

9　Roll to a rectangle and repeat steps 5–8 twice until all the fat is added. If the pastry becomes sticky at any time leave in the refrigerator for 10 minutes.
10　Repeat once more without the fat.
11　Use for vol-au-vents, Russian fish pie, sweet and savoury turnovers etc.

When flaky and rough puff pastry are cooked the fat melts and is taken up by the flour. The steam from the water in the pastry makes the pastry puff up and the layers set with the heat.

13 Scones, biscuits and cakes

Types of mixture

Scones, biscuits and cakes are made from flour, fat and liquid (usually milk or eggs). What makes them different is the amount of fat added and the method of mixing.

Rubbed-in mixture (up to $\frac{1}{2}$ fat to flour)

Fat and flour are rubbed together with the finger tips until the mixture is like fine breadcrumbs.

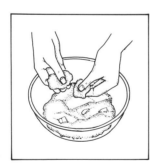

Melted mixture ($\frac{1}{2}$ fat to flour)

Fat, sugar and syrup are melted together.

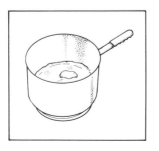

Creamed mixture (equal–$\frac{3}{4}$ fat to flour)

Fat and sugar are beaten together with a wooden spoon until light and fluffy. Then eggs are beaten in.

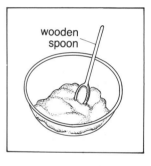

wooden spoon

Whisked mixture (no fat)

Eggs and sugar are whisked together.

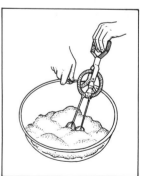

Scones, biscuits and cakes in our diet

Sugar

Most biscuits and cakes and some scones have a large amount of sugar added so eating them too often is not good for the teeth or the figure. It is sometimes possible to cut down the amount of sugar used and add dried fruits or other flavourings such as lemon or orange rind and juice or spices. You could also make savoury biscuits flavoured with herbs, cheese etc. Melted mixtures usually have the most sugar as they have syrup in as well.

Instead of putting icing on the top of cakes use fresh or dried fruits. Sprinkling with a little icing sugar also uses less sugar than making icing.

Fat

Scones, biscuits and cakes also contain a lot of fat. Whisked mixtures contain no fat at all, and rubbed-in and melted mixtures contain less than creamed mixtures.

Fibre

Use wholemeal flour or a mixture of white and wholemeal to add fibre. Try replacing some of the flour with porridge oats sometimes too, as this is another way of adding fibre, and add dried fruits like dates, raisins and apricots.

Questions

1 Most cakes and biscuits will be high in fat and sugar. You may be able to make them more nutritious by cutting down on sugar and by increasing fibre if you use wholemeal flour instead of white.
    In another recipe book find some biscuit and cake recipes. How could you change (adapt) the recipe to make them more nutritious?

2 When you buy cakes and biscuits you may be buying other ingredients besides the ones *you* would add. Collect wrappers from bought cakes and biscuits and list the ingredients. Write beside this the recipe you would use for the same dish. Which ingredients in the bought foods are additives (ingredients added just to change the colour, taste or keeping properties of the foods)?

Scones

The basic recipe is given here. Scones can be sweet or savoury, depending on the extra ingredients added (see suggestions below).

Scones (Rubbed-in-method)

Serve for tea, packed meals   Cook at Reg 7
                               220° C
Serve with low fat spread   Time 12–15 minutes
Makes 9

Ingredients

100 g wholemeal flour
100 g white flour
2 teaspoons baking powder (*or* 1 teaspoon bicarbonate of soda and 2 teaspoons cream of tartar *or* 1 teaspoon bicarbonate of soda and 1 teaspoon of cream of tartar and 150 ml sour milk)
40 g polyunsaturated margarine
150 ml skimmed milk

You could add any of these

Fruit scones

75 g dried fruit (e.g. currants, raisins, sultanas, cherries, dates)

Spicy scones

1 level teaspoon mixed spice

Cheese scones

50 g finely grated cheese

Herb scones

1 teaspoon dried herbs

Ham and parsley scones

25 g finely chopped ham
1 tablespoon chopped parsley

Apple and cinnamon scones

1 peeled and grated cooking apple
1 level teaspoon cinnamon

Method

1 Put the oven on. Grease a baking tray.
2 Rub the fat into the flour with the finger tips.
   Add enough milk to make a soft (not sticky)
   dough, mixing together with a knife.
3 Knead lightly together.
4 Roll out into a
   rectangle about
   1 cm thick and cut
   six 5 cm circles.

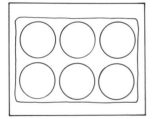

Re-roll and cut two.

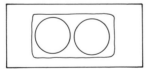

Make one from
remaining bits.

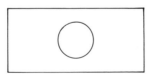

5 Place the scones on the baking tray and
   brush the tops with milk.
6 Bake 12–15 minutes until golden and risen.

Try a peanut filling for a change with savoury
scones. Chop, liquidise or food process 50 g
unsalted peanuts. Beat into 50 g low fat spread.

Biscuits

N.B. Most biscuit mixtures are soft when they
come out of the oven. Leave in the tin to cool
and go crisp.

Granola bars (Melted method)

Serve for tea, packed meals	Cook at Reg 4
	180° C
Makes 12 bars	Time 25 minutes

Ingredients

25 g flaked almonds
25 g hazelnuts
4 tablespoons vegetable oil
3 level tablespoons honey *or* golden syrup
50 g soft brown sugar
100 g porridge oats
25 g desiccated coconut
25 g sesame or sunflower seeds

Nuts and whole grain cereals can be bought at
health food shops. They also sell health food
bars, but you can make your own chewy version
with this recipe.

Method

1 Put the oven on. Grease an 18 cm square,
   shallow tin.
2 Chop the almonds and hazelnuts finely.
3 Put the honey or syrup, oil and sugar in a
   saucepan and warm gently.
4 Add all the other ingredients to the pan.
5 Press the mixture into the tin.
6 Bake until golden and set.
7 Leave to cool for 5 minutes. Mark into
   fingers.
8 Leave to cool in the tin.

Fruit slice (Rubbed-in method)

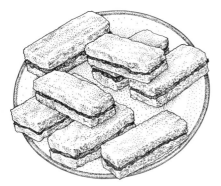

Figure 13.1

Serve for tea, packed meals	Cook at Reg 5
Makes 12 fingers	190° C
	Time 30–35 minutes

Ingredients

100 g wholemeal flour
100 g white flour
50 g soft brown sugar
125 g polyunsaturated margarine
200 g dates, raisins, apricots

Method

1 Put the oven on. Grease an 18 cm square, shallow tin.
2 Pour boiling water over the fruit and leave to soften.
3 Put the fat, sugar, and flour into a mixing bowl. Rub together with finger tips.
4 Press into a stiff paste.
5 Divide the paste into two. Press one piece into the bottom of the tin. Roll the other piece roughly to fit the top of the tin.
6 Drain the fruit and chop finely.
7 Spread the fruit over the biscuit mixture.
8 Cover with the rest of the mixture. Press down and level the top with a knife.
9 Cook 30–35 minutes until pale golden.
10 Cool slightly, then cut into fingers.

Wholemeal shortbread
(Rubbed-in method)

Serve for tea, packed meal	Cook at Reg 4
Makes 8 slices	180°C
	Time 25–30 minutes

Ingredients

75 g wholemeal flour
75 g white flour
100 g polyunsaturated margarine
50 g soft brown sugar

You could add any of these

Hazelnut shortbread

50 g hazelnuts
1 level teaspoon cinnamon

Cherry shortbread

50 g finely chopped glacé cherries
Finely grated rind of half a lemon

Cheese shortbread

50 g finely grated cheese
1 level teaspoon paprika

Method

1 Put the oven on. Grease a 20 cm flan ring and a baking tray.
2 Put the flour, sugar and fat into a mixing bowl and rub together with the finger tips.
3 Mix in the other ingredients.
4 Press the mixture into the flan ring on the baking tray.
5 Cook until dry looking, and slightly brown.
6 Cool slightly and mark into pieces.

Peanut butter cookies
(Creamed method)

Serve for tea, packed meals
Makes 20

Cook at Reg 4
180° C
Time 10–15 minutes

Ingredients

75 g polyunsaturated margarine
50 g peanut butter
100 g soft brown sugar
75 g wholemeal flour
50 g white flour

Method

1 Put the margarine, peanut butter and sugar together in a bowl and beat together (cream) with a wooden spoon until creamy.
2 Stir in the flour. Use your fingers to press together to form a soft dough.
3 Cut the dough into four pieces. Roll each piece to a sausage shape 20 cm long. Cut each piece into five.
4 Place the pieces on the baking tray and flatten with the back of a fork.
5 Bake until pale golden.
6 Cool on the tray for 10–15 minutes, before placing on a rack to go cold.

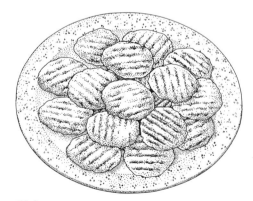

Figure 13.2

Banana cookies (Melted method)

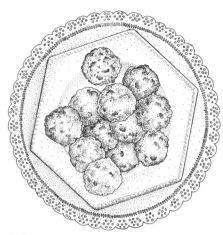

Figure 13.3

Serve for tea, packed meal
Makes 15

Cook at Reg 4
180° C
Time 15 minutes

Ingredients

100 g porridge oats
100 g sunflower seeds
1 tablespoon vegetable oil
2 tablespoons honey
1 ripe banana
1 egg

Method

1 Put the oven on. Grease a baking tray.
2 Grind the seeds and oats to flour in the blender or food processor.
3 Heat the oil and honey gently in a saucepan.
4 Beat the egg lightly. Mash the banana.
5 Mix the honey mixture into the seeds and oats.
6 Stir in the banana and egg.
7 Drop teaspoons of the mixture onto the baking tray, not too close together. Flatten slightly.
8 Bake until golden.

Fruit flapjacks (Melted method)

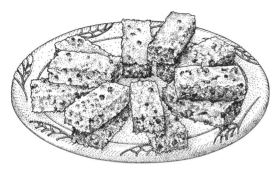

Figure 13.4

| Serve for tea, packed meal | Cook at Reg 4 180° C |
| Makes 12 fingers | Time 30–40 minutes |

Ingredients

200 g porridge oats
4 level tablespoons golden syrup
75 g demerara sugar
100 g polyunsaturated margarine
75 g dried fruit (e.g. currants, sultanas, raisins, dates, cherries, apricots)

You could add any of these

Spicy flapjacks

1 teaspoon ginger instead of or as well as the fruit

Peanut flapjacks

(Leave out the fruit)
50 g peanut butter instead of 50 g of the margarine
1 tablespoon unsalted peanuts roughly chopped, sprinkled on top

Method

1   Put the oven on. Grease an 18 cm square, shallow tin.

2   Put the margarine, sugar and syrup in a saucepan and heat gently until the sugar and margarine have dissolved.
3   Stir in the oats and fruit.
4   Press into the tin.
5   Cook until golden and set.
6   Leave to cool for 5 minutes. Mark into fingers.
7   Leave to cool completely before removing from tin.

Basic biscuit recipes
(Creamed method)

Serve for tea, packed meals	Cook at Reg 4 180° C
Serve savoury biscuits with cheese	Time 12–15 minutes
Makes 15	

Ingredients

75 g caster sugar
75 g wholemeal flour
75 g white flour
75 g polyunsaturated margarine
1 egg yolk

You could add any of these

Orange biscuits

Grated rind of an orange

Spicy biscuits

$\frac{1}{4}$ teaspoon cinnamon

Fruit biscuits

50 g currants or very finely chopped cherries or dates

Cheese biscuits

50 g finely grated cheese

Herb biscuits

1 teaspoon finely chopped dried herbs

Oat biscuits

Add 50 g porridge oats *instead of* 50 g of the flour
Add any of the flavourings above

Method

1 Put the oven on. Grease a baking tray.
2 Beat (cream) the margarine and sugar together with a wooden spoon until creamy.
3 Mix in the flour and any other flavourings.
4 Add enough egg to give a stiff dough.
5 Roll out 4 mm thick. Cut into circles with a 6 cm fluted cutter.
6 Place on the baking tray and cook 12–15 minutes.

Cakes

Treacle fruit buns
(One-stage method)

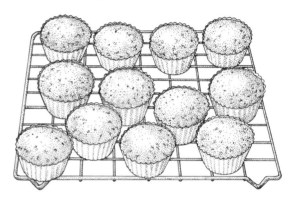

Figure 13.5

Serve for tea, packed meal
Makes 12

Cook at Reg 4
180° C
Time 15–20 minutes

Ingredients

150 g wholemeal flour
50 g polyunsaturated margarine
75 g dark soft brown sugar
1 tablespoon black treacle
50 g currants
75 g raisins or dates
2 rounded teaspoons baking powder
1 teaspoon mixed spice
1 teaspoon ground ginger
1 teaspoon cinnamon
100 ml skimmed milk

Method

1 Put the oven on. Put 12 paper cake cases in bun tins.
2 Put all the ingredients together in a bowl and beat well together.
3 Place teaspoons of the mixture in the bun cases. Bake until firm.

Banana fruit (or nut) loaf
(Rubbed-in method)

Serve for tea, packed meal	Cook at Reg 4
	180° C
Serve with low fat spread	Time 1 hour
Serves 4	

Ingredients

100 g wholemeal flour
100 g S.R. white flour
1 teaspoon baking powder
50 g margarine
50 g caster sugar
75 g raisins or sultanas *or* 50 g broken walnuts
1 egg
2 medium bananas
75 g golden syrup

Method

1 Put the oven on. Grease a 20 × 10 cm loaf tin.
2 Rub the margarine into the flour and baking powder until like fine breadcrumbs.
3 Add the sugar and fruit or nuts.
4 Mash the bananas and mix with the egg and syrup.
5 Pour into the dry ingredients and mix everything well together.
6 Pour into tin and bake until firm and golden.

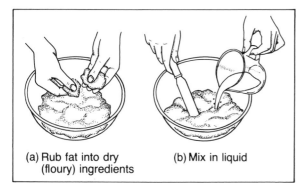

(a) Rub fat into dry (floury) ingredients   (b) Mix in liquid

Figure 13.6 Rubbed-in method

Cheese loaf (Rubbed-in method)

Serve for tea, packed meal, buffet	Cook at Reg 4
	180° C
Serve with low fat spread	Time 1 hour
Serves 4–6	

Ingredients

125 g wholemeal flour
100 g white flour
1 teaspoon baking powder
75 g firm low fat cheese
$\frac{1}{2}$ teaspoon dry mustard
1 teaspoon dried mixed herbs
1 egg
150 ml skimmed milk
Watercress and tomato

Method

1 Put the oven on. Grease a 20 × 10 cm loaf tin.
2 Grate the cheese finely.
3 Rub the fat into the flour and baking powder.
4 Mix in the cheese, mustard and herbs.
5 Add the egg and milk and mix together with a fork.
6 Spread in the tin. Bake until firm and golden.
7 Serve with watercress and tomato.

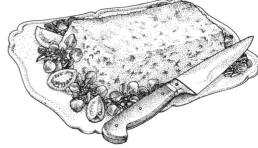

Figure 13.7

This loaf can also be made by the all-in-one method. Add an extra teaspoon of baking powder, put all the ingredients in a bowl and beat together.

Orange and cinnamon squares (Melted method)

Serve for tea, packed meal
Makes 12 squares

Cook at Reg 4 180° C
Time 30–35 minutes

Ingredients

50 g wholemeal flour
50 g white flour
$\frac{1}{2}$ level teaspoon bicarbonate of soda
$\frac{1}{2}$ level teaspoon cinnamon
50 g polyunsaturated margarine
25 g soft brown sugar
50 g golden syrup
1 rounded tablespoon orange marmalade
1 small orange
70 ml skimmed milk
1 egg

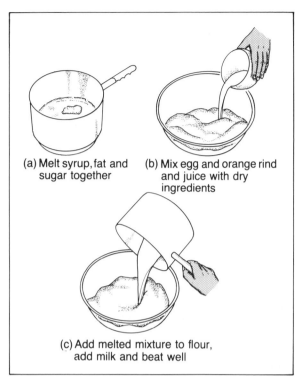

(a) Melt syrup, fat and sugar together

(b) Mix egg and orange rind and juice with dry ingredients

(c) Add melted mixture to flour, add milk and beat well

Figure 13.8 Melted method

Method

1 Put the oven on. Grease and line the bottom of an 18 cm square cake tin.
2 Scrub the orange. Grate the rind and squeeze the juice out.
3 Beat the egg lightly.
4 Place the flour and cinnamon in a bowl.
5 Place the margarine, syrup, marmalade and sugar in a saucepan and heat gently together until melted.
6 Add the egg, orange rind and juice and the melted mixture to the flour.
7 Put the milk into the same pan. Warm gently. *Do not* boil.
8 Pour over the bicarbonate of soda.
9 Beat the mixture until smooth with a wooden spoon. Beat in the milk.
10 Pour into the tin and bake until firm.

Lemon and date squares
(Creamed method)

Serve for tea, packed meal

Makes 15

Cook at Reg 5
190° C

Time 20–30 minutes

Ingredients

100 g polyunsaturated margarine
100 g soft brown sugar
2 eggs
2 tablespoons lemon curd
50 g dates
50 g walnuts
100 g wholemeal flour
1 level teaspoon baking powder

Method

1   Put the oven on. Grease a 25 × 15 cm shallow tin and line the bottom.
2   Chop the dates and walnuts.
3   Cream the margarine and sugar together with a wooden spoon until light and fluffy.

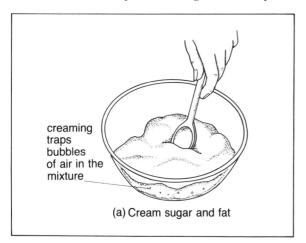

creaming traps bubbles of air in the mixture

(a) Cream sugar and fat

4   Beat the eggs lightly. Add to the creamed mixture a little at a time, beating well, so that mixture does not curdle. Beat in lemon curd.

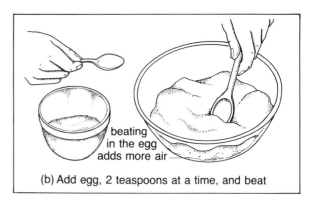

beating in the egg adds more air

(b) Add egg, 2 teaspoons at a time, and beat

5   Mix in the flour, one-third at a time, gently folding in with a metal spoon. Mix in the dates with the flour.

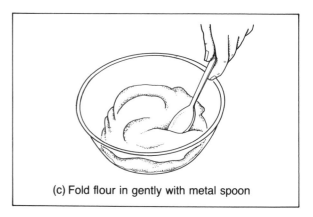

(c) Fold flour in gently with metal spoon

6   Mix to a soft dropping consistency — mixture should flick gently off the spoon. (Add a little water, if needed.)

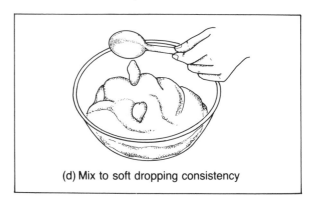

(d) Mix to soft dropping consistency

7 Spoon the mixture into the tin. Make the top level with a knife. Sprinkle with the walnuts.
8 Bake until springy. Test by pressing gently with your finger — it should not leave a mark.
9 Cool in the tin for a short time, then cut into squares.

Whisked sponge sandwich (Whisked method)

Serve for tea
Makes 8 slices

Cook at Reg 4
180° C
Time 15–20 minutes

Ingredients

75 g caster sugar
40 g wholemeal flour
35 g white flour
3 eggs
Jam or lemon curd to fill

Method

1 Put the oven on. Grease, line and flour two 15 cm round sponge tins.
2 Put the eggs and sugar in a bowl and whisk until thick and creamy. The mixture should leave a trail if dripped on the top.
3 Sieve the flour in, one-third at a time. Fold in gently with a metal spoon.
4 Pour the mixture into the tins and let it level off.
5 Bake until golden, and the mixture starts to shrink away from the sides.
6 Allow to cool slightly before turning out.
7 When cool spread with jam or lemon curd.

Because they do not contain any fat, whisked sponges will not keep for long without becoming dry. They are delicious eaten fresh. Any left-over dry sponge can be used in the bottom of trifles.

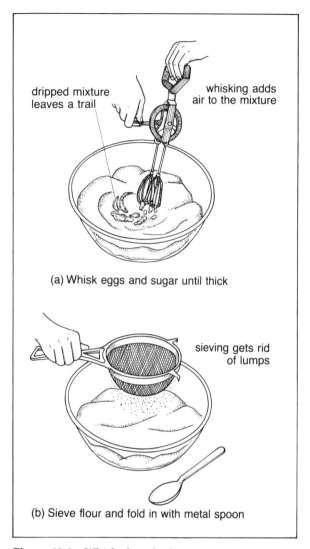

(a) Whisk eggs and sugar until thick

dripped mixture leaves a trail

whisking adds air to the mixture

sieving gets rid of lumps

(b) Sieve flour and fold in with metal spoon

Figure 13.9 Whisked method

Swiss roll (Whisked method)

Serve for tea
Makes 1 large roll or
9 individual rolls

Cook at Reg 7
220° C
Time 7–10 minutes

Ingredients

2 eggs
50 g caster sugar
50 g wholemeal flour
1 tablespoon warm water
Jam or lemon curd to fill
Extra caster sugar

Method

1 Put the oven on. Grease and line a
   20 × 30 cm Swiss roll tin.
2 Whisk the eggs and sugar together until
   thick and creamy (see previous recipe).
3 Fold in the flour gently, one-third at a time,
   and add the water.
4 Pour into the tin and let the mixture run
   into the corners.
5 Bake near the top of the oven until golden.
6 While the Swiss roll is cooking cut a sheet of
   greaseproof paper a bit bigger than the Swiss
   roll. Sprinkle with caster sugar. Have ready
   a sharp knife for cutting the edges and a
   knife for spreading.
7 Warm the jam slightly.
8 Turn the cake out onto the sugared paper.
   Remove the lining paper. Cut off the crisp
   edges (save these for a trifle).
9 Roll up the Swiss roll quickly, using the
   paper to help you. Hold for a few seconds.
10 Unroll. Spread with the jam. Roll up tightly.
11 Put on a rack and allow to cool.

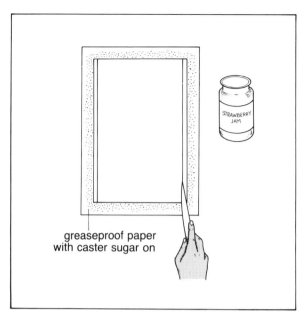

greaseproof paper
with caster sugar on

Figure 13.10   Trimming the edges

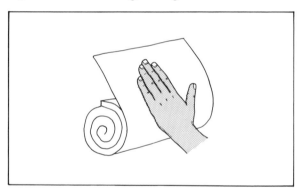

Figure 13.11   Rolling up

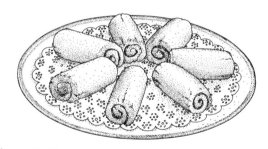

Figure 13.12

Individual Swiss rolls

Small individual Swiss rolls can be made.
1 Make and cook the mixture as before, but use a 35 × 15 cm tin. Cook 7–10 minutes, and be careful not to overcook. Turn out as before.
2 Cut into three across.
3 Spread each piece with jam and roll up lengthwise.
4 Cut each roll into three.

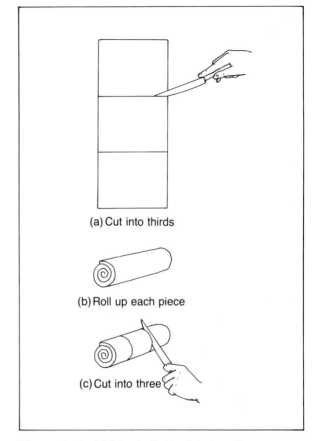

(a) Cut into thirds

(b) Roll up each piece

(c) Cut into three

Figure 13.13 Making individual Swiss rolls

14 Yeast mixtures

Bread in our diet

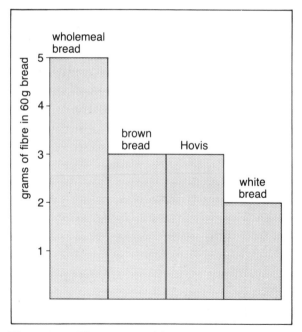

Figure 14.1 The amount of fibre in different kinds of bread (60 g is about 2 slices)

Bread forms a major part of our diet. It provides us with protein, and can be a good source of fibre as long as we choose the right type.

We should try to include more starchy carbohydrate and fibre in our diet and changing to wholemeal bread is one of the easiest ways to eat more fibre. Bread has fewer kilocalories (kilojoules) than cakes and biscuits, and wholemeal bread has fewer kilocalories than white. Bread also contains calcium and B vitamins.

Making bread

Bread is made from flour, yeast and liquid (usually milk or water). The yeast makes the bread rise and gives it a spongy texture. Sometimes fat, sugar or eggs are added, but these are not necessary. If large amounts of these are added you will have a rich bread dough, suitable mainly for sweet breads.

Yeast

This can be either fresh or dried. Dried yeast is tiny pellets of yeast which look like seeds and will keep for many months in the cupboard so that it is readily available when you want it. Dried yeast is more concentrated than fresh (about twice as strong).

Fresh yeast can be bought at the baker's and it

can be stored in the freezer for several months. It has a lemony smell and is crumbly.

Flour

The flour used in breadmaking should be *strong* flour. This is flour which comes from Spring wheat (for example Canadian wheat). Our climate is too wet to produce good bread flour. Strong flour gives a stretchy dough which will hold its shape well.

Proving

Bread takes quite a long time to make if you are going to knead it enough to make it rise evenly. It has to be left to **prove**, to give the yeast time to give off the carbon dioxide which causes the dough to rise — this makes the holes you can see. It is possible to shorten the time by adding a vitamin C tablet to improve the dough, and by giving it a really good kneading at the beginning.

This is what most bakers do to save time when producing large quantities of bread which will keep well. This method of making bread is called the *Chorleywood process* because it was developed at the Baking Research Association laboratory at Chorleywood.

The quick method for making bread is the one opposite.

Questions

1   Bread is called the 'staple' food in our diet. It is the food around which many of our meals are centred; as sandwiches, bread and cheese, toast for breakfast, for example. In other countries the staple food is different, for example in India it is rice. Why do you think this is? Find out what the staple foods are in other countries. Arrange them, in order, to show which provide the most nutrients in the diet.

2   Not all types of bread provide the same amount of nutrients. For example: Wholemeal bread, made from wholemeal flour, which contains 100% of the wheat grain has 9% fibre.

Other brown breads, made from brown flours, which contain 70–95% of the whole wheat grain have 5% fibre.

White bread, made from white flour which has nearly all the bran removed has 3% fibre. Some white bread has bran added to it, to replace the wheat bran which has been taken away.

Find out what types of bread are sold at your local baker's shop or supermarket. Arrange them in order to show which has the most fibre.

Bread — loaf or rolls

Serve for breakfast, tea, lunch, snacks
Serve with savoury or sweet spreads, for toasted snacks etc.
Makes one 400 g loaf or 8 rolls

Cook at Reg 7 220°C
Time 20 minutes for rolls
40 minutes for loaf

Ingredients

150 g strong white flour
150 g wholemeal flour
15 g polyunsaturated margarine
15 g fresh yeast or half a packet dried yeast (10 g)
About 200 ml warm water/skimmed milk
1 level teaspoon sugar
Half a 30-mg vitamin C tablet (you can buy these at the chemist's)
A little extra skimmed milk

Method

1   Put the oven on. Grease a baking tray and a polythene bag.
2   Put the flour in a bowl in a warm place. Try to keep everything gently warm as you are working, as the yeast needs warmth to

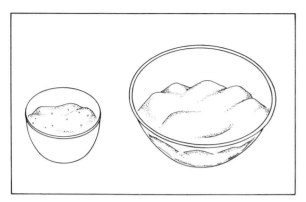

Figure 14.2   Fermenting. Put bowls of yeast and flour in a warm place (e.g. above the cooker, near a radiator, in the airing cupboard).

work. Too much heat will kill the yeast so do not overdo it.

3   Make the liquid warm by adding boiling water to the milk. Use 100 ml of each.
4   Put the yeast, sugar and milk in a bowl in a warm place until frothy. This will mean that the yeast is starting to give off carbon dioxide (ferment).
5   Rub the margarine into the flour until well mixed in.
6   Crush the vitamin C tablet up with a teaspoon. Add to the liquid.
7   Pour all the liquid into the flour.

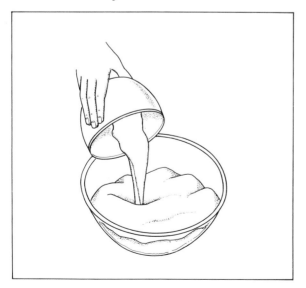

Figure 14.3   Mixing. Pour the yeast mixture into the flour.

8   Mix to a soft dough with a wooden spoon.
9   Turn onto a floured table and knead for at least 5 minutes to spread the yeast evenly.

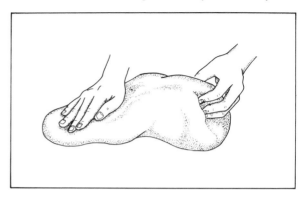

Figure 14.4   Kneading. Hold the dough with one hand while drawing the dough towards you with the other.

Kneading also helps to strengthen the gluten which is found in strong flour and helps the dough to become stretchy. Kneading can be done with an electric mixer which has a dough hook.

10   Shape the bread. For a loaf, pat to the shape of the tin and place carefully in the tin. For rolls, cut into eight pieces and shape. You could try any of the shapes in Figure 14.5.
11   Leave in a warm place to prove. Cover, if possible, with a greased polythene bag, greaseproof paper or damp teatowel. During proving the yeast ferments more and gives off carbon dioxide and alcohol which gives a characteristic smell. The bread should double in size (about 20 minutes).
12   Brush with milk.
13   Bake until golden brown and hollow sounding when tapped on the bottom.

Poppy or sesame seeds may be sprinkled on the top of bread before baking for a change.

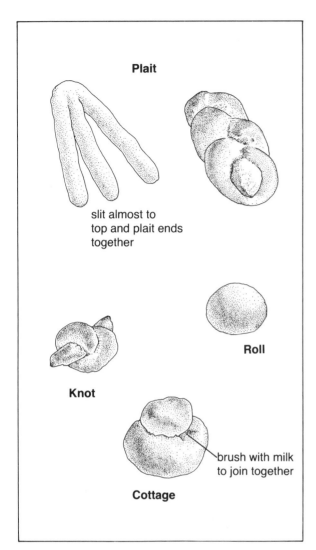

Figure 14.5 Bread roll shapes

Other types of bread

Other types of bread may be made using the same recipe but adding other ingredients.

Tea ring or currant buns

Add 150 g currants. Shape the currant buns into rounds and cook for 20 minutes on a greased baking tray, *or* press the tea ring into a greased ring mould and cook for 40 minutes.

Savoury breads

Tomato bread

Use tomato juice instead of milk. Add 1 teaspoon paprika with the flour. Make into rolls (cook 20 minutes) *or* make a large plait (cook 30–40 minutes on a greased baking tray).

Onion bread

Add a small finely chopped onion to the flour. Shape into a French loaf, cottage loaf or coburg. Cook 30–40 minutes on a greased baking tray.

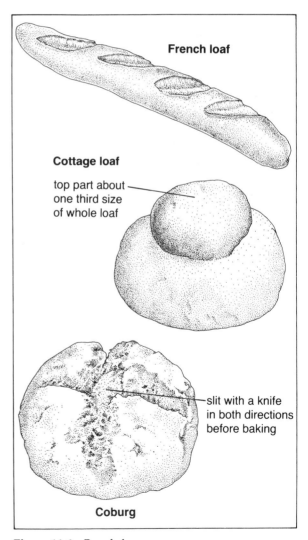

Figure 14.6 Bread shapes

Pitta bread

This is a flat bread with air trapped inside making a pocket which can be filled with hot or cold savoury fillings. It can be eaten as a snack meal, for a packed meal or with kebabs or other Greek foods.

Divide the dough into six. Knead each piece into a ball. Roll each ball to an oval measuring 30 cm down the centre. Sprinkle lightly with flour. Damp the edges by brushing with water. Fold each in half by bringing the top edge (further from you) over the bottom. Press the edges well together to seal. Bake on a greased baking tray for 20–25 minutes. Because this bread is not proved it remains flat.

Pizza

Make the bread as for loaf or rolls using half the recipe. Press into a 20 cm flan ring on a greased baking tray and leave in a warm place to prove. Prepare and put on any of the toppings as for Scone based pizza (see page 80). Bake 25–30 minutes.

15 Packed meals

Planning

There are times for most of us when we need food away from home, and it is cheaper or more convenient to take something with us. Planning a packed meal needs as much care as planning any other sort of meal.

A packed meal should:

(a) contain a variety of foods (and therefore a variety of nutrients);
(b) not have too much fat, sugar or salt;
(c) provide some fibre, e.g. wholemeal bread or pastry, vegetables, fruit;
(d) be easy to eat;
(e) be carefully packed so that it is not spoiled when carrying;
(f) include a drink.

Some suitable foods

The type of food for a packed meal will depend on who is going to eat it and where it is going to be eaten.

Choose from these groups

Filled wholemeal rolls or wholemeal pitta bread (see pages 145 and 148 and below)
Cheese loaf with fillings (see page 138 and below)
Individual pizzas (see page 80)
Individual quiches (see page 81)
Wholemeal pasties (see page 94)
Bran muffins with slices of cheese (see page 31)
Savoury filled scones (see page 132 and below)
Nutty Scotch eggs (see page 96)

Salads (see chapter 9) with cooked chicken pieces, ham, celery stuffed with cottage cheese, hard boiled eggs

Apple and date slices (see page 118)   } not too much of these
Wholemeal biscuits and cakes (see chapter 13)

Fresh fruit
Fresh fruit desserts (see chapter 10)
Yogurt

Drinks or soup (see chapters 7 and 11)

Some examples of packed meals

Packed meals for school lunch

Young children use up a lot of energy at school so include enough filling foods, which will also give some fibre, and some protein foods like meat, fish, or eggs or cheese. Calcium will also be needed so give milk drinks or foods containing cheese or yogurt. Pack in a lunch box or tin which will stand up to rough treatment. Include a fruit or milk drink or soup which can be carried in a flask.

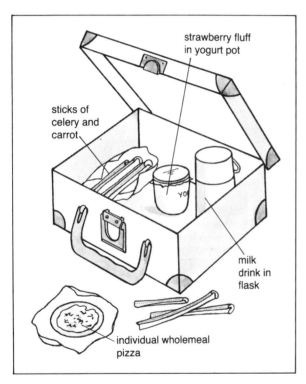

Figure 15.1   Packed meal for school lunch

Packed lunches for work

Choose a meal which can be eaten easily with the fingers. It may be possible to get a drink so it may not be necessary to include one. Think of the sort of work that the person does. Someone who sits down all day will not need foods to provide as much energy as someone who works on a building site. Think about how the person travels when packaging — someone travelling by train may want a slim box to slip into a briefcase.

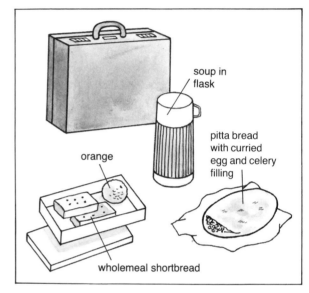

Figure 15.2   Briefcase meal in a slim sandwich box

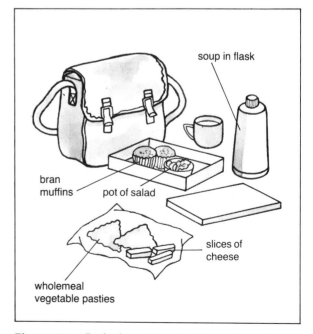

Figure 15.3   Packed meal for a building site worker

A packed meal for a coach or train journey

Food should be easy to unpack and eat. It should not make crumbs, or leave any litter. A thermos flask with a drink will be useful.

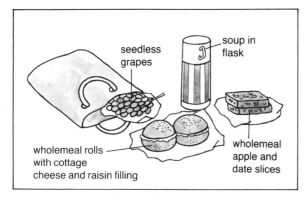

Figure 15.4 Packed meal for a train journey

A packed meal for a walking or cycling trip

When food has to be carried all day it needs to take up as little space as possible and should be packed so that it is light and does not squash. It should provide energy to keep the person going.

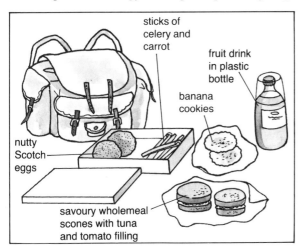

Figure 15.5 Packed meal for a walking or cycling trip

A packed meal for a journey by car

For a car journey a meal which needs knives, forks and spoons could be planned. There is no need to worry as much about crumbs, and drinks could be carried in bottles or flasks.

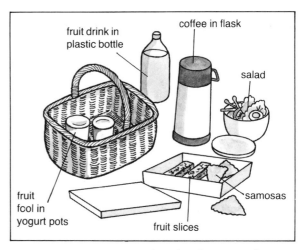

Figure 15.6 Packed meal for a family on a car journey

Fillings for packed meals

These fillings can be used for wholemeal rolls, cheese loaf, pitta bread etc.

Fillings for packed meals should include some protein food — cheese, eggs, meat, fish or vegetables. They should not be too fatty. Make them moist by adding chutney, mayonnaise, relishes, and there should be no need for any extra fat on the bread. Spread well to the edges to avoid dryness. Add salad foods for extra vitamins.

Some fillings to try

1 Cottage cheese with:
   chopped red pepper and watercress *or*
   raisins *or*
   chives
2 Slices of Edam cheese and apple
3 Mashed hard boiled egg with:
   tomato and bean sprouts *or*
   chopped ham *or*
   chopped celery, curry powder and chopped almonds
4 Cold scrambled egg with curry powder and peas
5 Minced chicken and ham with a little mayonnaise or chutney
6 Corned beef, mashed with chutney
7 Tuna and chopped tomato

8   Meat or nut loaf with lettuce and cucumber
9   Peanut butter with chopped cucumber, carrot, celery, onion
10 Left-over cooked vegetables made into a paste in the food processor

Questions

1   Fillings for sandwiches, rolls or pitta bread can become boring. Try to think of six other fillings, including two suitable for a vegetarian, two which are low fat, and two suitable for a slimmer.

2   Suggest something for a lunchbox for a 5-year-old to replace the following:
a bag of crisps
a chocolate biscuit
a sausage roll

16 Dishes for young children

Young children's needs for food change very quickly from birth onwards. For more information about children's needs for food see *Families and Child Development*.

Infancy (up to 1 year)

First weeks

For the first weeks of life a baby needs only milk. Human breast milk is the best start in life a mother can give her baby:
1 It contains just the right nutrients for the baby.
2 It is at just the right temperature.
3 The mother passes on immunity from certain diseases (the baby is not so likely to catch them).
4 The milk is sterile (free from germs).
5 It is easily digested by the baby.

Sometimes it is not possible to breast feed, and bottle feeding will be fine as long as the instructions for making up bottle milk are carried out properly. Feeding bottles and teats must be sterilised and just the right amount of milk powder used. Some parents have put extra powder in the feed thinking it will be good for

the baby, but it puts a strain on the baby's kidneys and can be *dangerous*. Cow's milk should not be given to babies under 6 months.

Baby (2–3 months)

Extra iron and vitamin C are needed as the baby grows. This can be given in juices. It is not a good idea to put sweet things in a baby's dummy as this can cause tooth decay even before the baby's teeth can be seen, and you do not want the baby to get too fond of sugar.

Weaning (4 months onwards)

Weaning means gradually introducing solid foods. Before 3 months a baby's kidneys and digestive system are not developed enough for solid food, but by about 4 months milk on its own will not give enough nutrients for growth. Solid foods should be introduced gradually, and will need to be sieved or puréed so that the baby will not choke when they are swallowed. Some first solid foods might be:
>   rusks or ground cereals in milk
>   puréed vegetables, meat, fish, fruit
>   cooked egg yolk
>   egg custard

Do not add sugar or salt. Sugar now will only encourage children to like sweet things all their lives and this will be bad for teeth and health. Too much salt will put a strain on the kidneys.

Some foods like rusks, toast or apple (peeled) will help the teeth to develop.

It is much cheaper to use a food processor, liquidiser, sieve or baby food grinder and make your own baby foods from foods the family is eating than to buy pots of baby food. Some bought baby foods contain a lot of sugar and salt so if you do use them look for the salt and sugar free ones.

Young children (1–5 years)

As children grow they will need especially:

protein — for growth
calcium — for bones and teeth
flouride — for teeth
iron — for red blood cells

Do not give too many fatty foods, as a build-up of cholesterol can start in the arteries from very early on. Encourage the eating of crunchy, high fibre foods.

Meals should look attractive to encourage children to eat. If they do not like something do not force it. Leave it and try again at another time. Try serving foods in different ways too. Milk, for calcium and vitamin D, can be served as flavoured milk drink, milk puddings, cheese sauce etc. This should be whole milk not skimmed, unless the doctor advises otherwise, to help children meet their kilocalorie (kilojoule) needs.

Young children have small appetites, so little and often is the best rule — with regular meal times. Often food is refused if sweets and snacks are eaten between meals so avoid giving these. They may cause tooth decay and weight problems.

Avoid giving too many convenience foods as these contain artificial additives, e.g. colouring in squash, jelly, ice lollies.

Suitable dishes

Breakfast

Cereal with milk   *or*
Yogurt   *or*
Fresh fruit

Eggs (boiled, poached, scrambled (see page 29)
    or
Small piece of grilled or poached fish   *or*
Small rasher of grilled bacon, tomato

Wholemeal toast with low fat spread and yeast
    extract or a little marmalade or jam

Milk   *or*
Fruit juice (see pages 27, 124)

Midday/Evening

Fish, e.g. Fish mornay (see page 72)
        Fish pie (see page 73)
        Fish and cheese crumble (see page 74)
or
Cheese e.g. Savoury supper dish (see page 36)
or
Meat, e.g. Chicken and ham loaf (see page 50)
        Chicken fricassee (see page 50)
or
Eggs, e.g. Egg mornay (see page 85)

Fresh fruit   *or*
Mousse   *or*
Yogurt   *or*
Fruit fool (see page 122)

Fruit juice   *or*
Milk

For a lighter meal

Wholemeal sandwiches (see page 149) *or*
Omelette

Fruit   *or*
Yogurt

Milk   *or*
Fruit juice

N.B. Whole nuts and peas should not be given

to children under 5 as they can become stuck in the throat or nose.

Questions

1 If you had young children and a grandparent or friend wanted to give them sweets, what would you say to explain the problems without offending them?

2 Make up the home-made version of some canned or bottled babies' foods. You can use a liquidiser, food processor or baby food grinder to make the foods into a purée. Compare the taste, texture, cost and time taken to make each. You may not think baby foods have much flavour, but remember, a baby will not be used to strong tasting foods like you. Make a list of the ingredients on the label of the bought food. Which do you think would be the best choice for a baby, the home-made or bought variety?

3 Ice lollies are popular with young children, but they also contain a lot of sugar, colourings and flavourings. It is possible to make your own ice lollies using plastic moulds, freezing them in the freezer or ice-making compartment of a refrigerator. You could use fresh orange or other fruit juices to make the ice lollies. Can you think of any other types of lolly that you could make?

Recipes for young children

In addition to the dishes mentioned above, these recipes are also suitable for young children.

Baked stuffed liver

Serve for main meal, for children
Serve with potatoes

Cook at Reg 5
190°C
Time 45 minutes

and a fresh vegetable
Serves 4

Ingredients

300 g liver
250 ml water + half a stock cube
2–3 tablespoons packet veal stuffing
2–3 slices lean bacon

Method

1 Put the oven on. Grease a 750 ml casserole dish.
2 Wash the liver. Remove the skin and gristle.
3 Cut in thin slices, and small pieces.
4 Put in the casserole dish.
5 Sprinkle the stuffing on top.
6 Boil the water and dissolve the stock cube.
7 Pour stock so that it comes three quarters of the way up the liver.
8 Remove any fat from the bacon. Spread over the liver.
9 Cook until the liver feels tender.

Meat loaf

Serve for main meal, for children
Serve with tomato sauce and potato, or salad
Serves 4

Cook at Reg 4
180°C
Time 45 minutes

Ingredients

400 g minced beef
100 g wholemeal bread
Half a stock cube
1 small onion
100 ml water
1 egg
Pinch pepper
1 teaspoon savoury sauce, e.g. Worcestershire
Browned breadcrumbs (raspings)

Method

1 Grease a 15 cm loaf tin. Coat with browned breadcrumbs.
2 Peel and grate the onion.
3 Make fresh breadcrumbs from the bread.
4 Mix the beef with the rest of the ingredients to a soft dropping consistency.
5 Press into the tin.
6 Cover with foil or greaseproof paper and cook until firm.
7 Serve with tomato sauce (see page 113).

Hickory dickory mouse

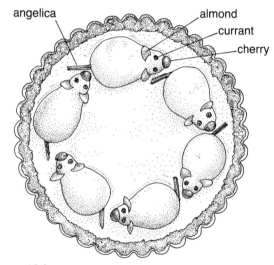

angelica   almond
            currant
            cherry

Figure 16.1

Serve for sweet, for children
Serves 4

Ingredients

50 g polyunsaturated margarine
8 digestive biscuits
Medium can pears in unsweetened juice
1 packet blancmange
50 g granulated sugar
500 ml milk
Currants, cherries, angelica, almonds to decorate

Method

1 Grease a 20 cm flan dish.
2 Crush the biscuits in the liquidiser, food processor, or with a rolling pin between two sheets of greaseproof paper.
3 Melt the margarine. Stir in the biscuit crumbs. Press round the sides and bottom of the flan dish.
4 Make blancmange following the instructions on the packet. Pour onto the biscuits. Chill.
5 Drain pears.
6 Place the pears on to the blancmange when set, and decorate as in Figure 16.1.

Children will often not drink milk. This recipe and the next give ways in which to tempt a child to take milk.

Mandarin delight

Serve for a sweet, for   Cook at Reg 3
children   170°C
Serves 4   Time 20 minutes

Ingredients

50 g dried milk
50 g rice
50 g caster sugar
2 eggs
Small can mandarin oranges in unsweetened juice
Angelica to decorate

Method

1 Mix 500 ml water with the dried milk in a saucepan.
2 Add the rice and boil gently together until creamy and thick.
3 Cool.
4 Separate the eggs. Add the yolks to the rice.
5 Cover the bottom of a casserole dish with mandarin oranges keeping a few back for decoration.

6 Pour the rice mixture over the fruit.
7 Whisk the egg whites until so stiff that you can turn the bowl upside down without the mixture falling out.
8 Whisk in 25 g caster sugar. Fold in 25 g caster sugar.
9 Pile the meringue mixture over the rice. Brown lightly in the oven for 20 minutes.
10 Decorate with mandarin oranges and angelica before serving.
11 Serve hot or cold.

Orange dessert

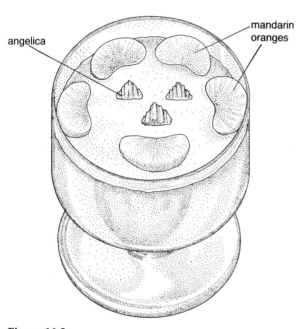

Figure 16.2

Serve for sweet, for children
Serves 6

Ingredients

Small can evaporated milk
250 ml water
Large can mandarin oranges in unsweetened juice
2 tablespoons lemon juice
3 rounded teaspoons gelatine
Angelica to decorate

Method

1 Dissolve the gelatine in the juice from the fruit.
2 Make up to 475 ml with water.
3 Put in the fridge or freezer to half set.
4 Whisk the milk and lemon juice into the jelly with the mandarins, saving some for decoration.
5 Pour into individual glasses and leave to set.
6 Decorate as below.

17 Reheated dishes

Food is too expensive to throw away and left-over food can often be made into tasty dishes. Using left-overs is called réchauffé (reheated) cookery. Care is needed when using left-over foods to cook them thoroughly to kill bacteria, as food can easily be re-infected even if the bacteria have been killed when the food was first cooked.

Points to remember

1 Cool left-over food as quickly as possible and keep, covered, in the refrigerator. Any bacteria present will multiply if the temperature is right.
2 Use the food within 48 hours at the longest. It is best used as soon as possible.
3 Do not reheat food more than once or you will give bacteria a chance to become active.
4 Left-overs can be dry so add cold sauce, stock or gravy and mix with other cooked foods.
5 It is easy to overcook food when cooking for the second time so cover with pastry, egg and breadcrumbs, sauce or potato.
6 Add extra flavourings, e.g. herbs, as some of the flavour may have been lost when the food was first cooked.

7 Serve reheated food immediately so that bacteria do not get a chance to multiply.
8 Serve reheated foods with fresh fruit, vegetables or salad as many of their vitamins will have been lost in the first cooking.
9 Do not give reheated foods to infants or invalids as they are less digestible than freshly cooked foods and may have lost vitamins B and C.
10 Finely mince or chop foods to cut down cooking time.

Some dishes using left-over food

Fish

Kedgeree (see page 74)
Fish pie (see page 73)

Meat

Curry (see page 52)
Stuffed pancakes (see page 86)
Rissoles (see below)

Bread

Summer pudding
Bread and butter pudding (see page 160)

Cake

Bakewell tart (see page 160)
Trifle

Question

How could you use the following leftover
ingredients?
Cooked potatoes
Cheese
Rice
Stewed apple

Rissoles

Serve for main meal	Cook at Reg 4
Serve with tomato	180° C
sauce (see page 113),	Time 35 minutes
potatoes, fresh vegetable	
Serves 4	

Ingredients

100 g cooked meat
100 g potatoes
Pinch black pepper
1 level teaspoon chopped parsley or herbs
1 teaspoon Worcestershire sauce
1 egg
Dried breadcrumbs
Parsley to garnish

Method

1 Put the oven on. Grease a baking tray.
2 Scrub, peel and cook the potatoes in boiling
   water for 20 minutes or until tender.
3 Mince the meat.
4 Mash the potatoes.

5 Mix the mince, potatoes, pepper, herbs and
   Worcestershire sauce together. Cool.
6 On a floured table and with floured hands
   make into a roll. Divide into eight portions.

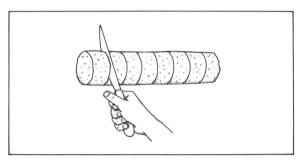

Figure 17.1   Shaping rissoles

7 Coat with beaten egg, then breadcrumbs (see
   page 96).
8 Place on the baking tray. Cook for 15
   minutes. Turn over. Cook for another 20
   minutes until golden.

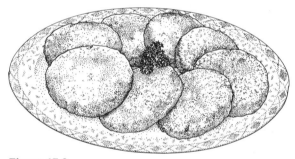

Figure 17.2

Bread and butter pudding

Serve for pudding
Serves 4

Cook at Reg 4
180° C
Time 45–60 minutes
or Microwave
(see below)

Ingredients

6 thin slices dry wholemeal bread
30 g polyunsaturated margarine
75 g dried fruit (currants, sultanas, apricots, raisins)
30 g caster sugar
2 eggs + 1 extra yolk
500 ml milk
Powdered nutmeg

Add some sliced banana for a change.

Method

1 Put the oven on. Grease a casserole dish.
2 Spread the bread with margarine. Cut the crusts off. Cut into triangles.

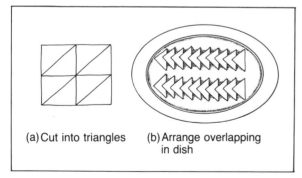

(a) Cut into triangles   (b) Arrange overlapping in dish

Figure 17.3 Arranging the bread

3 Arrange half the bread in the dish, overlapping the pieces.
4 Sprinkle with all the fruit and half the sugar.
5 Arrange the rest of the bread on top.
6 Sprinkle with the rest of the sugar.
7 Beat the eggs and milk together.
8 Pour over the bread. Sprinkle the top with nutmeg.
9 Cook until set and golden brown.

To microwave:

Cook uncovered in the microwave for 3 minutes.
Press the bread down.
Leave to stand for 5 minutes.
Cook uncovered 5 minutes.
Leave to stand 15 minutes.
Cook, uncovered, 3–5 minutes until set. Remove from the oven.
Leave to stand 5 minutes.
Brown the top under the grill.

Bakewell tart

Serve for sweet, tea, packed meal
Serve with custard for a pudding
Serves 4

Cook in Microwave
Time 4 + 4 minutes

Ingredients

For the pastry

50 g wholemeal flour
50 g white flour
50 g margarine
Water to mix

For the filling

37 g polyunsaturated margarine
50 g caster sugar
50 g left-over cake
50 g ground almonds
1 egg
Vanilla essence
1 tablespoon jam

A few cherries to decorate

This recipe has been specially developed for cooking in the microwave cooker.

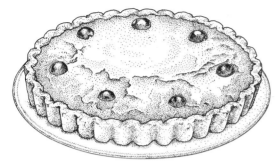

Figure 17.4

Method

1 Make the pastry by rubbing the fat into the flour until like fine breadcrumbs. Add enough water to make a stiff dough.
2 Roll out to fit a 20 cm china or glass flan dish.

3 Microwave the pastry case for 4 minutes.
4 Break the cake into crumbs. Chop the cherries into quarters.
5 Separate the egg. Whisk the white until you can turn the bowl upside down without it falling out.
6 Beat the sugar, margarine, almonds, cake crumbs, egg yolk and 4 drops vanilla essence together with a wooden spoon, or use a food mixer.
7 Fold the egg white in gently.
8 Spread the jam in the bottom of the pastry case.
9 Spread the mixture over.
10 Place the cherries on the top, pressing into the mixture.
11 Microwave 4 minutes.
12 Allow to cool and sprinkle lightly with icing sugar (as the top will not brown in microwave cooking).

18 Convenience foods

Convenience foods are foods which have been processed and packaged to save time and energy in preparation and cooking. They also make it possible to have foods when they are not in season.

Advantages of convenience foods

1 Convenience foods are quick and easy to prepare.
2 They can be stored in the cupboard or freezer for times of emergency, e.g. when the weather is too bad to go out, or someone is not well enough to shop.
3 They are suitable for times when there is not much cooking equipment, e.g. camping, caravan, self-catering holidays.
4 There is very little waste.
5 Some foods have added vitamins, e.g. some cereals have B vitamins added.

Disadvantages of convenience foods

1 Most convenience foods contain a lot of additives. Frozen foods contain the least. Additives are not needed by the body and can even make some people ill. They are added to provide colour or flavour or to help preserve the food. Always look at the labels on food as they have a list of the ingredients with the ones there are most of at the top. That way you can tell whether you are buying more food or more additives.
   For more on additives see the section on labelling in the book *Home and Consumer* in this series.
2 Convenience foods often contain a lot of fat, sugar and salt. Again, a look at the label will tell you if these are high on the list.
3 They do not contain much fibre (except for canned baked beans, kidney beans, sweetcorn).
4 Some nutrients may have been lost when the food was processed.
5 Convenience foods are often more expensive than the fresh food or home cooked dish.
6 Portion sizes are often small.
7 They hardly ever taste the same or as good as the fresh food.

Cooking with convenience foods

Types of convenience foods which are useful in cooking are:

Frozen foods

Fruit, vegetables, meat, fish, pastry, dough, ready-meals, pies, cakes, cold sweets, ice cream.

Canned foods

Fruit, vegetables, pulse vegetables in sauce (e.g. baked beans), soup, milk puddings, fish, meat, baby foods.
Some salt and sugar free fruit and vegetables can be bought.

Dehydrated (dried) foods

Potatoes, vegetables, soup, pot foods, meat dishes, packet mixes for cakes, bread, puddings. Some of these foods are Accelerated Freeze Dried (AFD) which is a mixture of freezing and drying.

Recipes

As long as you do not rely on convenience foods all the time there is no reason why they should not sometimes be a part of meals. Some dishes in this book use convenience foods for all or part of the recipe to save time and energy in preparation.
   As well as the recipes below see:
Fruit flan (page 120)
Mandarin flan whip (page 121)
Sunflower shortcake (page 123)
Strawberry fluff (page 122)

Questions

1   Make a list of the convenience foods you have in the cupboard or freezer at home. Suggest a meal which could be made from these.

2   Collect labels from a range of convenience foods. Divide them into groups:
high in additives
medium amount of additives
few additives

3   Make up a home-made version of a bought convenience food dish. Organise a testing panel to compare appearance, taste, texture, cost, time, and ingredients of the home-made and bought versions. Which did your panel prefer?

Country fish dish

Serve for main meal
Serve with fresh vegetables
Serves 4

Ingredients

4-serving packet of potato mix
400 g fresh or frozen cod
4-serving packet of thick country vegetable soup
150 ml skimmed milk
50 g firm low fat cheese

Method

1   Grease a shallow casserole dish.
2   Grate the cheese.
3   Cook the fish with 2 tablespoons of the milk, on a covered plate, over a pan of boiling water for 10–15 minutes until tender (or microwave covered for 5–10 minutes).
4   Pour off the liquid and make up to 400 ml with water. Add the soup. Put in a saucepan, bring to the boil and simmer for 20 minutes.
5   Make up the potatoes as on the packet, adding enough milk to make them creamy. Fork or pipe the potato round the edges of the dish.
6   Remove any bones and skin from the fish and break up with a fork. Stir into the soup.
7   Pour the fish into the middle of the potatoes.
8   Sprinkle with the grated cheese. Grill until golden brown.

Lasagne

Serve for main meal
Serve with salad
Serves 4

Cook at Reg 5
190° C
Time 30 minutes

Ingredients

6 sheets of lasagne
60 g polyunsaturated margarine
60 g wholemeal flour
500 ml skimmed milk
150 g firm low fat cheese
400 g can minced steak
Pinch nutmeg
Pinch black pepper
Pinch cayenne pepper
1 tomato

Watch out for the lasagne which does not need cooking first. This will save time so you can leave out step 3.

Method

1   Put the oven on. Grease a shallow casserole dish.
2   Grate the cheese. Wash and peel the tomato and slice thinly.
3   Cook the lasagne in boiling water for 12 minutes. Drain. Rinse with boiling water, and keep warm.
4   Make a roux sauce with the margarine, flour and milk (see page 114).
5   Remove from the heat and stir in the black pepper, cayenne and nutmeg and the cheese, saving a little of the cheese for the top.
6   Arrange layers of the lasagne, mince and sauce ending with the sauce.
7   Sprinkle the cheese on top.
8   Bake until golden. Put the tomato slices on top for the last 10 minutes.

Tuna and mushroom with rice

Serve for main meal
Serve with salad or fresh vegetable
Serves 3–4

Ingredients

500 ml packet mushroom soup
200 g can tuna
150 g long grain rice
1 egg
2–3 tomatoes

Method

1   Hard boil the egg. Cool.
2   Cut the egg into slices or quarters. Peel and slice the tomatoes.
3   Cook the rice in boiling water until tender (about 20 minutes). Drain.
4   Make the soup following the instructions on the packet, but only use half the water.
5   Flake the tuna with a fork. Add to the soup. Heat gently through for 4–5 minutes.
6   Arrange the rice round the edge of the dish. Pour the sauce in the middle.
7   Garnish with slices of tomato and egg.

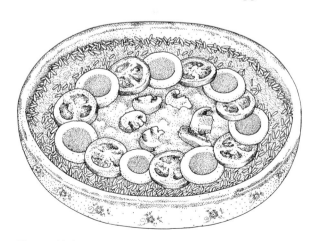

Figure 18.1

Apricot tart

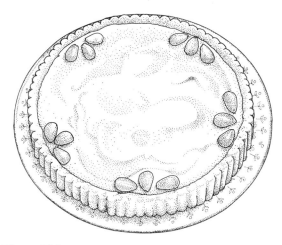

Figure 18.2

Serve for sweet, buffet
Serves 4

Ingredients

150 g digestive biscuits
25 g granulated sugar
50 g polyunsaturated margarine
400 g can apricots
10 g gelatine (just less than a packet)
3 tablespoons hot water
Halved blanched almonds to decorate

Method

1 Grease a 20 cm flan dish.
2 Crush the biscuits with a rolling pin between two sheets of greaseproof paper or in a polythene bag, or use a food processor.
3 Melt the margarine in a saucepan with the sugar. Stir in the biscuit crumbs.
4 Press the crumbs round the sides and bottom of the flan dish. Put in the refrigerator.
5 Sieve, liquidise or food process the can of apricots.
6 Dissolve the gelatine in the water by standing the bowl in a saucepan of simmering water (or microwave for 30 seconds).
7 Mix into the apricot purée.
8 Pour into the biscuit case and set in the refrigerator.
9 When set, decorate with almonds.

19 Coping with special needs

A special diet is sometimes needed when some part of the body is not working as it should. Usually a doctor, or the dietitian at a hospital, will give guidance on what foods to avoid, or eat more of, on a special diet.

Foods during illness

When someone is ill (an **invalid**) or recovering from an illness (**convalescent**) they may especially need foods containing protein, to replace or build body tissue; calcium, if bones have been broken; and iron, if there has been bleeding. If they have a very poor appetite and cannot eat very much it is important to provide these nutrients in liquids, e.g. soup or broth (for protein and iron), fruit juice (for vitamin C), glucose drinks (for energy) and milk (for protein and calcium). See the Egg flip recipe on page 125. All body processes need water. Because we continually lose water through excretion, everyone, including the sick, needs water. Plenty of non-alcoholic drinks are the easiest way to have this.

Once the patient is out of bed and moving around again the appetite usually returns and solid foods will be needed:

1 Serve meals that contain a variety of foods and therefore nutrients.
2 Choose foods that are easy to digest.
3 Serve small portions, as appetite will still be small and energy needs low.
4 Avoid fatty foods (e.g. fried foods, oily fish, pork, rich pastry, cakes and biscuits) as they are not easily digestible.
5 Avoid very strongly flavoured foods. The smell and flavour can make people feel worse.
6 Make meals look attractive, to tempt the appetite.

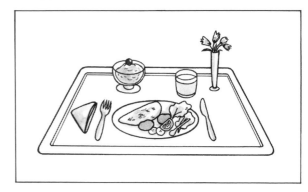

Figure 19.1 A meal to serve for an invalid

7 Serve at the right temperature, e.g. hot dishes should be hot, not lukewarm, so that they taste as appetising as possible.

8 Do not use left-overs in case of infection from bacteria. Use only very fresh food.

9 Include foods that contain fibre, to prevent constipation. Eating fresh fruit helps.

Suitable dishes

Some dishes to serve might be:

Breakfast

Cereal, porridge with milk
Fresh orange juice or an orange
Poached, boiled or scrambled eggs with toast (see page 29)
Wholemeal toast
Milk drink (e.g. wake-up breakfast drink, page 27)

Main meals

Fish mornay (page 72)
Fish pie (page 73)
Egg mornay (page 85)
Omelette (page 35)
Baked stuffed liver (page 155)

Fresh vegetables (chapter 9)

Fresh fruit salad (page 122)
Fruit fool (page 122)
Strawberry fluff (page 122)
Apple snow (page 123)
Bread and butter pudding (page 160)

Fruit or milk drink (chapter 11)

Anaemia

Anaemia is caused when the body does not get enough iron. This may be because of loss of blood through illness or surgery, through not eating enough of the foods containing iron, or may occur in adolescence when menstruation starts.

The doctor will probably prescribe iron tablets, but the following foods contain iron and serving these will also help:

> red meats, especially liver, heart, kidney,
> pulse vegetables, e.g. peas, soya beans (these would be particularly useful for a vegetarian)
> bread, flour, some breakfast cereals, black treacle, dried fruits

It is a good idea for everyone to make a point of having one meal rich in iron each week.

Iron is not used easily by the body, but vitamin C helps the body to absorb it, so it is a good idea to serve foods containing vitamin C with the foods containing iron, e.g. baked stuffed liver with a fresh green vegetable, sardine and tomato sandwiches. Liver and kidneys are not liked by many people, but you can mix them with other meats, e.g. with minced beef when making spaghetti bolognese.

Diabetes

Diabetes is a disease people suffer from when their bodies do not produce enough insulin to deal with the sugar in their blood. The doctor will prescribe insulin injections or tablets or just a special diet to cope with this. The insulin will balance the glucose (sugar) in the blood which mainly comes from foods rich in carbohydrate. If diabetics are given too little insulin and /or too much carbohydrate their blood sugar level will rise too high (hyperglycaemia). If they are given too much insulin and/or not enough carbohydrate their blood sugar level will fall too low (hypoglycaemia). Regular meals are important for a diabetic to keep the blood sugar level at a happy medium.

Diabetic diets

Diabetics are usually given a list of foods and their carbohydrate content, so that they can plan meals with the amount of carbohydrate and fibre recommended by the doctor.

Some carbohydrate foods are absorbed more slowly than others. To keep the blood sugar level steady it is best to have most of the carbohydrate allowed from the slowly absorbed carbohydrate foods. These are:

    pulses, e.g. peas, beans
    most fruit
    wholemeal bread and crispbread
    whole grain and bran breakfast cereals
    potatoes (especially if the skins are eaten)
    brown rice and wholemeal pasta
    most vegetables (especially if eaten raw)

These foods will also provide fibre in the diet.

Carbohydrate foods which are quickly absorbed and cause a sharp rise in the blood sugar level include sugar, biscuits, cakes, sweets. Diabetics should save these foods for 'emergency' treatment during an attack of hypoglycaemia or for during very energetic exercise.

Because carbohydrate foods also help to put on weight, it is important for diabetics not to have too many fatty foods, and to take plenty of exercise.

Low salt diets

The proper name for salt is **sodium chloride**, and it is the sodium part of salt which may cause problems in the diet. Normally the body can balance the amount of sodium in it by altering the amount which is excreted through the kidneys. If the kidneys or heart are not working properly salt can collect in the body. The body then holds extra water which can sometimes be seen in puffy ankles and hands. High salt intakes may cause blood pressure to rise (hypertension). It may then be necessary to have a low salt diet. It would be a good idea for everyone to cut down the amount of salt in their diet to help prevent this from happening.

To reduce salt in the diet:
1 Avoid convenience foods (look for anything with 'sodium' on the label and you will see just how much salt we eat).
2 Eat as much fresh food as possible and do not add salt when cooking.

3 Avoid using baking powder and bicarbonate of soda.
4 Remove the salt cellar from the table (or if you cannot give it up altogether make the holes smaller).
5 Add spices, herbs and other flavourings to dishes instead of salt.

Low fat diets

A low fat diet may be needed if there is some problem with digestion or absorption of fat by the body, or following a heart attack.

It is almost impossible to cut fat out completely as it is present in so many foods, but it is possible to eat less of it. It would help reduce the possibility of heart disease if we all cut down the amount of fat we eat.

To reduce fat:
1 Grill or boil food instead of roasting or frying.
2 Trim off all the fat you can see from meat.
3 Eat poultry or fish in place of red meats.
4 Use cornflour for thickening casseroles instead of frying the meat or vegetables in fat and mixing with the flour, *or* toss the meat in flour and add stock.
5 Skim fat off meat dishes.
6 Cook meat on a trivet so that fat drains off.
7 Replace full cream milk with skimmed milk.
8 Replace hard cheeses with cottage or low fat firm cheese.
9 Replace cream with natural yogurt.
10 Use low fat spreads in place of margarine or butter.
11 Leave out the fat used for spreading bread when making sandwiches and use just a moist filling instead.
12 Read the labels on packaged foods and avoid those containing fat.

Food allergies

Some people have an allergic reaction when they eat certain foods. This may result in a rash, headaches, puffiness of the face or wrists, sickness, diarrhoea or feeling unwell. Once the food causing these symptoms has been removed from the diet the symptoms disappear.

Milk allergy

Some people, especially some young children, are allergic to cows' milk. It can cause an eczema type of skin reaction, diarrhoea and sickness. It is possible to use goats' milk instead of cows' milk.

Allergy to additives

Some of the additives used in bought foods can cause an allergic reaction, e.g. over-activity and behaviour problems in young children. It is often difficult to work out exactly what is causing the problem as there are so many additives in bought foods. Additives such as preservatives and colourings now have an E number which must be shown on the label, e.g. tartrazine, E102, is a yellow colouring, found in many foods, to which some people have an allergic reaction. This is used in soft and fizzy drinks and ice lollies, packet dessert topping, fruit pie filling, canned vegetables, bought cakes etc.

We could all try to avoid allergies to food additives by:
(a) looking at the labels on packaged foods and avoiding those with too many additives;
(b) looking at a copy of *E for Additives** to find out more about the E numbers, what they stand for and which allergies they may cause.

Allergy to gluten

Gluten is formed from proteins found in wheat, oats, rye and barley when they are mixed with water. An allergy to gluten can cause coeliac disease which causes the intestines to become damaged so that little food can be absorbed. It is not easy to avoid gluten as it is contained in bread, biscuits, breakfast cereals, pasta, cakes, gravy powder etc. All these foods have to be avoided and it is possible to buy special gluten free flour for baking. It is necessary to read food labels carefully to avoid any wheat products and to be careful when eating out.

Questions

Now you know a little more about special diets try these.
1   Choose a midday meal for someone:
    (a)   recovering from flu;
    (b)   with a sore mouth, e.g. after having a tooth out;
    (c)   with anaemia.
    Explain why you have chosen each dish. Draw a diagram to show how you would serve the meal in part (a) to make it attractive to the patient.
2   Plan a packed meal suitable for a diabetic.
3   Choose 6 recipes from this book which are low in salt and show what has been used in place of salt to make the dish tasty.
4   Choose 6 recipes from this book which are low in fat. Write down any changes you think may have been made to the recipe to make it low in fat.
5   Collect some food labels from bought foods. Make a list of the E numbers shown. Find out why these additives have been included and what allergies they might cause.

* Maurice Hanssen, *E for Additives*, Thorsons, 1984.

20 Entertaining

There may be times when you want to provide food for friends for different occasions. Try to serve a variety of dishes and make the food look good by having different colours and textures. What you choose will depend on the time of day, the age and number of people, the occasion and the amount of money you are able to spend.

Recipes for all the dishes mentioned can be found in this book. Use the contents or the index to help you find them.

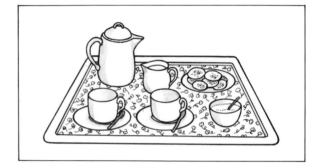

Figure 20.1 Serving coffee

Morning coffee

(Or when you are just having friends round at any time.)
Serve:
A drink — coffee or fruit or milk drink
Savoury or sweet biscuits or cake or Bran muffins
Savoury or sweet scones
Small slices of pizza

Include something savoury and something sweet.

A meal

Serve:
A starter
A main course
A sweet
A drink, e.g. coffee

Read chapter 2 to remind yourself of things to consider when planning a meal.

High tea

High tea is usually eaten at about 6 o'clock as one of the main meals of the day.
Serve:
A cooked dish, usually a complete meal in itself which does not need anything adding, e.g.
Savoury supper dish, Crisp tuna casserole, Risotto, Chicken fricassée, Spaghetti bolognese, Moussaka, Lasagne, Fish mornay, Fish pie, Fish and cheese crumble, Kedgeree, Vegetable pie
or
Something with a salad, e.g. Chicken and ham loaf, Savoury flan, Pizza, Quiche, Wholemeal pasties, Lentil and walnut loaf, Nutty Scotch eggs

Some sort of cake or biscuit
A cold sweet

A drink

Tea

Serve:
Savoury or sweet scones
Small slices of Pizza or Quiche
Bran muffins with slices of cheese
Cheese loaf with filling

Biscuits or cakes

Yeast mixtures, e.g. wholemeal (filled) rolls, Tea ring or Currant buns

Buffets

Serve foods which can be easily eaten with the fingers, or with a fork or spoon only.
Individual pizzas
Individual quiches
Cheese loaf
Samosas
Nutty Scotch eggs
Small wholemeal pasties
Savoury scones

Salads

Fresh fruit salad
Cheesecake
Fruit flan
Mandarin flan whip
Sunflower shortcake

Biscuits, cakes

A drink

For children's parties similar foods would be suitable, but serve in small portions and make the decorations suitable for children (see chapter 16).

21 Food preservation

Food is preserved so that it can be kept after the time when it would otherwise have gone bad. All foods go bad because they contain micro-organisms, e.g. bacteria, which multiply, (*micro* means very very small) and enzymes, e.g. those which make an apple go brown. Foods are also attacked from the air by moulds and yeast. You may sometimes see such moulds on bread or cheese.

To preserve food we must remove the conditions which let the bacteria and moulds grow, by:

(a) removing moisture, i.e. dehydration (drying);
(b) reducing the temperature, i.e. freezing;
(c) excluding air and sterilising (giving a very high heat treatment), i.e. bottling, canning;
(d) adding ingredients which stop the action of the organisms, such as vinegar, salt, sugar, i.e. pickles, jams.

The food must be sealed well to stop other micro-organisms from getting in.

Jam making

1 The jars must be prepared by washing, drying and sterilising in the oven on a baking tray covered with newspaper for 30–40 minutes at Reg 6, 200°C.

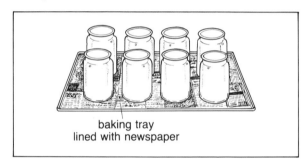

baking tray
lined with newspaper

Figure 21.1 Sterilising the jars

2 The fruit is softened and sterilised by cooking in water in a large preserving pan.

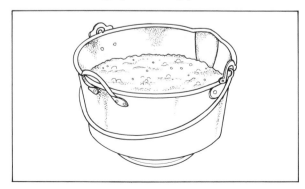

Figure 21.2 Softening the fruit in a preserving pan

Fruit contains in its cell walls a gum-like substance called **pectin**. This makes the jam set so the fruit must be simmered long enough for the pectin to be let out of the fruit. Some fruits have more pectin than others. Fruits with good amounts of pectin are:

> blackcurrants
> redcurrants
> damsons
> gooseberries
> bitter oranges
> lemons
> cooking apples

Fruits with a fair amount of pectin are:

> plum
> apricots
> raspberries
> blackberries

Fruits with poor amounts of pectin are:

> strawberries
> cherries
> pears

Sometimes fruits are mixed, in jams, when one of the fruits is low in pectin, e.g. blackberry and apple, strawberry and gooseberry.

3 Sugar is added to stop yeasts growing in the jam and to help it set. Jam should contain 40% fruit and **60% sugar**, but the amount you can add depends on the sort of fruit and the amount of pectin. After the fruit is softened it should be tested for pectin.

Testing for pectin

(a) Take 1 teaspoon of juice free from seeds and skin. Place in a cup or glass and allow to cool. Add 3 teaspoons of methylated spirit

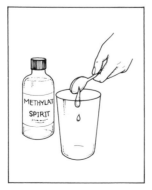

(b) Shake gently and leave for 1 minute

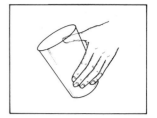

(c) Pour into another container and look at the clot that forms.
If you have a good clot add 700 g sugar to 400 g fruit.

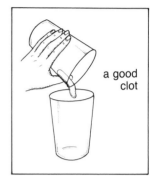

a good clot

If you have a fair clot add 400 g sugar to 400 g fruit.

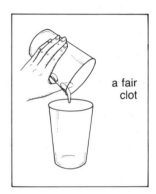

a fair clot

If you have a poor clot you will need to add more pectin by adding lemon juice or another fruit (cooked first) which is rich in pectin or the juice of a fruit which is rich in pectin.

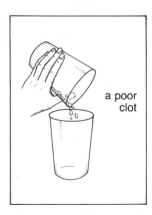

a poor clot

It is possible to buy pectin (e.g. Certo), but this is more expensive and gives a 'gummy' jam.

4 Once the sugar is added the jam can be boiled quickly until ready to set.

Testing for set

Remove the jam from the heat while testing, or it may overcook.

Wrinkle test

Put a little jam on a cold plate and allow to cool. Push with the finger. If it wrinkles it is ready to set.

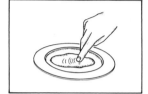

Temperature test

A sugar thermometer can be used to take a reading. (Keep the thermometer in boiling water until ready to use — it will crack if it is cold.) When the jam is ready to set it will reach 105°C (221°F).

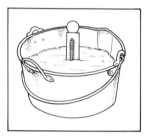

Flake test

Dip a clean wooden spoon in the jam. Allow to cool slightly, then let the jam run gently off the edge. If it comes off in wide flakes, it is ready. If it pours off, it is not.

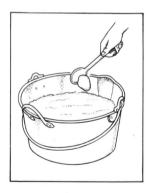

5   Turn off the heat and remove any scum which floats to the surface with a wooden spoon. A knob of margarine stirred into the jam will help the scum to float to the surface.
6   Use a jug to pour the jam into the jars. Fill to the top.
Be careful as the jam will be *very hot.*
7   Place a waxed circle touching the jam. Allow to cool.
8   When cool put a circle of cellophane over the top of the jar. Dip the cellophane in water

on one side to allow you to stretch it over the top, dry side down, and secure with a rubber band.
9   Label with the type of jam and date.

Faults in jam making

Jam may crystallise (go sugary) if:
(a)   it was not boiled for long enough;
(b)   it was overcooked;
(c)   too much sugar was added;
(d)   there was not enough acid (from the fruit or lemon juice) in the jam.

Jam may grow mould on the top if:
(a)   the fruit was over-ripe;
(b)   not enough sugar was used;
(c)   air has got into the jars because they were not sealed properly.

Jam may ferment (go fizzy) if:
(a)   it was not boiled for long enough to set;
(b)   not enough sugar was used;
(c)   poor fruit was used.

Question

It is possible to buy low-sugar jams. These may have additives in them to help to keep the jam for longer. Find a label for a low-sugar jam with these additives and list the ingredients. How else could low sugar jams be prevented from going off? How would you decide whether you wanted a jam high in sugar, high in additives, or one that might not keep so long? (You could spread jam more thinly to cut down on the sugar!)

Marmalade making

This is done in exactly the same way as jam, but the fruit needs boiling for longer to soften. Lemon juice is usually needed to give a set.

Jelly making

Jellies are like jam, but without the solid fruit. After the fruit is softened, as for jam, it is dripped through a jelly bag.

The bag should not be squeezed or the jelly will be cloudy. The juice is then returned to the pan, tested for pectin and finished as for jam.

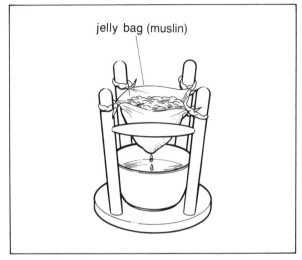

jelly bag (muslin)

Figure 21.3 Jelly making. An upturned stool is a good place to tie the jelly bag.

Freezing

To freeze food it must be stored at a low enough temperature to stop micro-organisms from growing, i.e. −10 to −20°C (5°F). When the food is thawed some micro-organisms may become active again so do not re-freeze.

Vegetables need to be blanched to slow down the activity of the micro-organisms so that they do not lose their colour and flavour.

To blanch vegetables

1 Turn the freezer to its coldest setting.
2 Prepare the vegetables.
3 Bring a large saucepan of water to the boil.
4 Put 400 g of the vegetables at a time into a wire basket.

5 Boil for 2–5 minutes, depending on the type of vegetable.
6 Lift the basket out and plunge into ice cold water or hold under the tap until cold.

Sample blanching times

Runner beans (cut into 2 cm lengths) 2 minutes
Brussels sprouts 4 minutes
Carrots (cut) 3 minutes
Corn on the cob (small) 5 minutes

Packaging

Food for the freezer should be packaged to cut out the air, e.g. in polythene bags, plastic tubs. Allow room for liquids to expand.

Place in the coldest part of the freezer. Freezing may take 6–7 hours.

Pickling

Fruit and vegetables can be preserved in vinegar or brine (salt water). They are first covered with salt or salt water for a few hours to stop the growth of bacteria and draw out some of their water so that they are crisp. They are then packed into jars and covered with cold spiced vinegar.

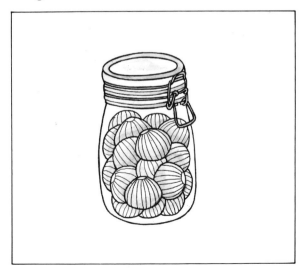

Figure 21.4 Pickled onions

To make spiced vinegar

Ingredients

500 ml vinegar
4 teaspoons pickling spice (cloves, peppercorns, dried chillies, cinnamon, ginger etc.)

Method

1 Heat the vinegar to just under boiling point with the spices. Do not let the vinegar boil rapidly as it will smell unpleasant and the fumes can remove paint.
2 Strain and cool.

  (*Or* put the spices in the cold vinegar and leave for 2 months.)

Chutneys

Fruit and vegetables are sterilised by boiling to a thick jam-like mixture. Vinegar and spices help to stop the growth of bacteria.

  It does not matter if the fruit is under-ripe for chutneys and they are a good way of using up gluts of fruit like green tomatoes and apples.

Drying

Herbs are the only foods to be dried at home. Pick herbs when they are about to flower. Wash, tie in bundles and dry in a warm place (e.g. the airing cupboard) or over the bars of the oven at Reg 6, or 200°C, until they feel dry. They can also be dried in the microwave cooker. Place on a piece of kitchen paper and microwave for 1 minute. Shake the paper and continue doing this until the herbs feel dry. Once dry they can be crushed with a rolling pin.

Quick recipes

Most recipes for preserves take a long time to make. The recipes here have been adapted so that they can be made in the microwave cooker which is quicker. Use a large bowl to give the mixture room to rise up when cooking — about 2 or 3 times as large as the amount of jam.

Green tomato or apple chutney

Makes 1½ kg

Cook in Microwave

Ingredients

600 g green tomatoes *or* apples *or* a mixture of both
300 g sultanas *or* raisins
150 g onions
2 teaspoons salt
1 teaspoon ground ginger
½ teaspoon cayenne pepper
200 g brown sugar
600 ml malt vinegar

Method

1 Prepare the jars as for marmalade on page 177.
2 Peel the onions and apples. Remove the cores from the apples. Chop the onion, tomatoes or apples or put through a mincer or food processor.
3 Place in a large bowl with the pepper, salt, ginger, vinegar and sultanas. Cover with cling film (make a hole in it). Microwave for 15 minutes or until pulpy.
4 Add the sugar and microwave for 50–55 minutes or until you have a jam-like mixture.
5 Fill the jars. Cover as for jam.

Three-fruit marmalade

Makes 2–3 kg

Cook in Microwave
Read the section about jam making (page 172)
before trying this recipe.

Ingredients

2 medium lemons
2 medium grapefruit
2 medium oranges
850 ml boiling water
2 kg sugar (preserving or granulated)

Method

1 Prepare the jars. Put a little water in each.
   Heat in the microwave for 2–3 minutes one
   at a time. Pour the water out and turn
   upside down to drain.
2 Wash and dry the fruit. Cut in half and
   squeeze out the juice. Save.
3 Remove the pith and pips from the fruit. Tie
   these in a piece of clean muslin.
4 Shred the peel. This can be done in the food
   processor. It may be fine or coarse.
5 Place the juice, bag of pips and pith, and
   peel with one-third of the water in a large
   mixing bowl. Soak for 1 hour.
6 Add the rest of the water. Cover the bowl
   with cling film, making two slits in it so that
   it does not balloon.
7 Cook in the microwave for 20 minutes if you
   cut the peel finely, 25–30 minutes if it was
   coarse.
8 Uncover and stir in the sugar. Cook,
   uncovered for 25–30 minutes or until setting
   point is reached. Stir every 5 minutes.
9 Leave in the bowl until a skin forms, then
   fill the jars.
10 Cool and cover as for jam.

Apple jam

Makes 680 g

Cook in Microwave

Ingredients

500 g cooking apples
550 g granulated sugar
1 tablespoon lemon juice

Method

1 Prepare the jars. Put a little water in each.
   Heat in the microwave for 2–3 minutes one at
   a time. Pour the water out and turn upside
   down to drain.
2 Wash, peel, core and slice the apples. Put
   them in a large bowl. Add the sugar. Do not
   mix. Heat uncovered in the microwave for 10
   minutes
3 With an electric mixer or wooden spoon beat
   the apples and sugar until well mixed.
4 Microwave for another 10 minutes.
5 Stir in the lemon juice.
6 Cool and pour into jars.
7 Cover, seal and label (see page 174).

22 Food and hygiene

To avoid becoming ill through food poisoning, care is needed when buying, storing and preparing food.

Buying food

1 Buy from shops which look and smell clean and appear to have a quick turn-over of goods.
2 Make sure the assistants handle the food properly, e.g. any damage to their skin must be covered, unwrapped meat, pastries and cakes should be picked up with tongs, hair should be covered or tied back.
3 Check that there are no animals in the shops.
4 Check the date stamps on food. Date stamps tell you when a food should be sold by.
5 Be especially careful when buying food from market stalls. It should be undamaged.
6 Food should be properly wrapped and sealed where possible. Avoid buying foods with damaged wrapping.

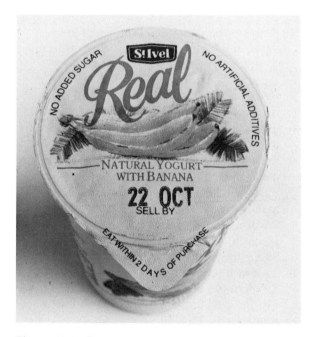

Figure 22.1 Date stamp on a carton of yogurt

Storing food

1 Rotate foods, i.e. put the new foods you have just bought to the back and bring the old ones forward to use first.

2 Store perishable foods in a cool place, preferably in the refrigerator.

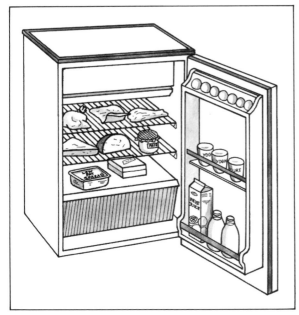

Figure 22.2   Perishable foods should be stored in the refrigerator.

3 Store root vegetables in a dry, airy place, e.g. a vegetable rack.

4 Store dry goods like flour in covered containers in a dry, dark place. Biscuits and cakes should be stored separately or the biscuits go soft.

5 Store bread in a ventilated bin (i.e. one with holes in).

6 Store raw meat separately from cooked meat.

7 Keep all food covered when working to protect from flies. Use polythene bags, cling film, foil, lids etc.

8 Cool left-over foods quickly, put in the refrigerator and use within 24 hours.

Preparing food

Personal hygiene

1 Before starting to cook, tie hair back, wash hands and scrub nails.

2 Wash hands after handling raw meat, visiting the toilet or putting rubbish in the dustbin.

3 Do not cough or sneeze over food.

4 Make sure that any breaks in the skin are covered.

5 Wear a clean apron.

6 Do not taste foods and then put the spoon back in. Drip food to be tasted onto a teaspoon for tasting.

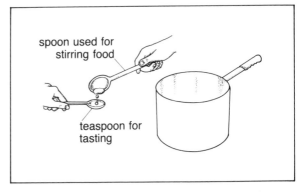

Figure 22.3   Tasting

Kitchen hygiene

1 Use hot soapy water for washing-up and change it often. An egg cup of bleach in the water should make sure that things are safely washed. Rinse, if possible, in hot water. Use only clean teatowels, or leave to dry in a rack.

2 Rinse dishcloths well in bleach and leave them in the air to dry.

3 Keep separate cloths for washing-up, cleaning the floor and for cleaning the dishes of pets.

4 Keep a separate set of dishes for pet food. Animals should be kept out of the kitchen.

5 Keep work surfaces and floors clean. Make sure they are made of cleanable materials and are free from cracks.

6 Keep waste bins covered and empty them often (at least once a day).

7 Keep nappy buckets out of the kitchen. They can be kept in the bathroom.

8 Use a disinfectant down the sink to keep water in the U-bend fresh smelling.

9 Avoid using chipped dishes.

Glossary of cooking terms

To **bake blind** To bake a pastry case without any filling. Greaseproof paper and baking beans or foil are used to hold the pastry on the bottom of the flan ring or dish while cooking.

To **baste** To spoon hot liquid over a food during cooking to keep it moist, e.g. basting meat with hot fat during roasting.

To **blanch** To put food into cold water and bring just to boiling point, then to plunge into cold water, e.g. almonds are blanched to remove their skins. Vegetables can be blanched before freezing, by putting them into boiling water for a few minutes, then into cold water, to prevent discolouring.

To **blend** To mix together a dry and a liquid ingredient. The cold liquid is added gradually and the mixture stirred to prevent lumps forming, e.g. cornflour and milk are mixed for a blended sauce.

Bouquet garni A small bunch of herbs tied together in muslin, used to flavour soups and stews, and removed before serving.

To **braise** To cook meat or fish on a bed of vegetables, with a little liquid, in a dish with a tight fitting lid. The dish is finished off by roasting with the lid off.

Consommé A very thin, clear soup.

To **cream** To work one or more ingredients with a wooden spoon until smooth and creamy, e.g. margarine and sugar are creamed together when making cakes.

Croûtons Bread, cut into small squares, or shapes fried or toasted, and usually served with soup.

Crudités Raw vegetables, often cut into thin strips, eaten with savoury dips.

To **dice** To cut food into small cubes.

To **flake** To break up food, e.g. fish, with a fork.

Forcemeat Stuffing, e.g. sage and onion forcemeat is served with pork.

Fricassee A white sauce with chicken, rabbit or veal.

Garnish A decoration on savoury dishes, e.g. sprigs of parsley on a pie, lemon butterflies on fish.

Glaze A clear jelly made from arrowroot and fruit juice or jam used on fruit dishes to keep them moist.

Hors-d'oeuvre The first course of a meal (French for 'outside the main work'), e.g. soup, pâté, prawn cocktail.

To **knead**   To work a dough lightly with the knuckles, as for bread, or with the finger tips, as for shortbread.

Mirepoix   A mixture of vegetables on which to put meat to braise (see above for braising).

Offal   The internal organs of an animal, e.g. liver, kidneys, heart.

Panada   A thick sauce for binding ingredients together, e.g. sauce for holding fish cakes together.

To **par-boil**   To partly cook by boiling, then finish off by another method, e.g. potatoes can be par-boiled, then roasted.

Pâté   A paste made from fish, meat or liver with flavourings.

To **poach**   To cook in liquid in an open pan with enough liquid to come at least half way up the food, e.g. poached eggs.

Pulses   Dried peas, beans and lentils.

Purée   A smooth pulp obtained by pressing vegetables or fruit through a sieve or by liquidising or food processing them.

Raspings   Very fine browned breadcrumbs used for coating foods. They can be made by drying bread in the oven and crushing with a rolling pin.

Réchauffé   Reheated.

Roux   A mixture of fat and flour cooked together for sauces, e.g. white sauce.

To **sauté**   To toss food in fat in a saucepan to add flavour and to start to cook it. This stage can often be left out to cut down on fat.

Seasoning   Salt and pepper added to dishes to improve flavour. The use of too much salt should be discouraged.

To **sieve**   To press food through a wire mesh to break it up or remove lumps.

To **simmer**   To cook slowly in liquid which is only just boiling. Bubbles should rise gently and just pop on the top.

To **skim**   To remove the top layer from a liquid usually with a spoon, e.g. the scum which rises when making jam is skimmed off. Milk may have the cream skimmed off to cut down the fat content.

Starter   See *hors-d'oeuvre*.

To **strain**   To pour off the liquid from ingredients, e.g. rice is strained before serving. This may be done through a special spoon with holes in, a colander or sieve.

Tepid   Warm. Two parts of cold liquid and one part of boiling will give a tepid liquid.

Zest   The outer coloured skin of citrus fruits (e.g. oranges, lemons). This contains the flavour. The white pith under the skin is bitter and not used. To remove the zest of a lemon peel the skin off finely or grate the rind.

Answers to pasta quiz on page 57

(a)   Macaroni (used in milk puddings, cheese sauce)
(b)   Vermicelli (used in soups)
(c)   Cannelloni (stuffed with meat sauce)
(d)   Ravioli (stuffed with meat and served in sauce)
(e)   Tagliatelli (served in meat or cheese sauce)
(f)   Lasagne (served with meat and cheese or white sauce). Lasagne verde is spinach flavoured lasagne and is green.
(g)   Spaghetti (served with meat or tomato sauce)
(h)   Pasta shells (pasta is made into various novelty shapes)

Index

In this index, recipes are listed both alphabetically and by their main ingredients. Dishes which are good sources of fibre, calcium, iron and certain vitamins (nutrients of which a shortage may be experienced) are additionally indexed under these nutrients.